B.O.O.B.S.

A BUNCH OF OUTRAGEOUS BREAST-CANCER SURVIVORS

TELL THEIR STORIES OF COURAGE, HOPE, & HEALING

Compiled & Edited by Ann Kempner Fisher

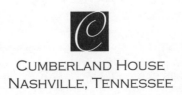

CUMBERLAND HOUSE
NASHVILLE, TENNESSEE

B.O.O.B.S.
PUBLISHED BY CUMBERLAND HOUSE PUBLISHING INC.
431 Harding Industrial Drive
Nashville, Tennessee 37211

Scripture quotations marked (KJV) are taken from the King James Version. Scripture quotations marked (NAB) are taken from the New American Bible with Revised New Testament and Revised Psalms © 1991, 1986, 1970 Confraternity of Christian Doctrine, Washington, D.C., and are used by permission. Scripture quotations marked (NIV) taken from The Holy Bible, New International Version. Copyright © 1973, 1978, 1984 International Bible Society. Used by permission of Zondervan Bible Publishers. Scripture quotations marked (NKJV) are taken from the New King James Version. Copyright © 1982 by Thomas Nelson, Inc. Used by permission. All rights reserved. Scripture quotations marked (NRSV) are from the New Revised Standard Version of the Bible, copyright © 1989 by the Division of Christian Education of the National Council of the Churches of Christ in the USA. Used by permission. All rights reserved.

Cover design: James Duncan Creative
Text design: Lisa Taylor

Library of Congress Cataloging-in-Publication Data
Fisher, Ann Kempner.
    B.O.O.B.S. : a bunch of outrageous breast-cancer survivors tell their stories of courage, hope, and healing / compiled and edited by Ann Kempner Fisher.
        p. cm.
    ISBN-13 978-1-58182-523-7 (paperback)
    ISBN-10 1-58182-385-1 (hardcover)
    1. Breast—Cancer—Patients—United States—Biography. I. Title: BOOBS II. Title: Bunch of outrageous breast-cancer survivors tell their stories of courage, hope, and healing. III. Title.
    RC280. B8F565 2004
    362.1'96994'0092—dc22

                                                                            2004003846

Printed in Canada
2 3 4 5 6 7 8 — 11 10 09 08

B.O.O.B.S.

In loving memory of

Marianne Bardoul Star
Ann Brett
Mary Drew
Virginia Van Valzah
Lucy Ann Russo
Cassandra Benton

CONTENTS

ACKNOWLEDGMENTS

We are forever indebted to Harold Benjamin, the founder of The Wellness Community, for his vision to provide a safe haven, free of charge, to cancer patients and their families and friends. We feel extremely fortunate for the enormous contribution he has made— and continues to make—to our lives.

Our deepest thanks to the staff of The Wellness Community– Atlanta for their compassionate guidance through the highs and lows of cancer diagnosis and treatment. They offered a "lifeline" of hope, courage, and strength in our quest to be survivors. Without their help to regain our wellness, we could not have undertaken this project.

We are blessed to have Carolyn Helmer at the helm, as Executive Director of The Wellness Community–Atlanta. We are thankful for her tireless efforts to keep our "community" a welcome and nurturing place.

Our appreciation to Dede Malpass, the facilitator of our breast-cancer group, for crying along with "her girls" when we shared our tearful moments and joining in our laughter as we found humor amidst adversity.

There are a number of special people who generously donated their time and talent to The Wellness Community educational programs and facilitated our healing. Tallulah Lyons for Exploring Dreamwork, Bobbie Spivey Fink for T'ai Chi, Edna Bacon for Recovery through Art, Heather Reed for Interactive Yoga, Merrilee Stewart for Stress Reduction to Enhance the Immune System, and Jill Hall, a cancer survivor, for Meditation and Survivorship. Thank you, one and all.

Every writer needs an editor, and we thank our literary editor, Ann Kempner Fisher, for making the details of numerous drafts bearable—we came to realize she was "heaven sent." She molded a diverse group of women into writers of their unique stories. Her editorial skill and creative guidance helped our written words reveal the inner strength, insight, and inspiration it took for each of us to survive. Ann shared her enthusiasm for the book with novelist, Jackie Miles, who suggested Ann "agent" the book to her publisher, Cumberland House Publishing.

To Jim Anderson, Mark Jefferson, and Rick Hirsch, our deepest thanks for sharing our enthusiasm and counseling us in legal matters.

Sheryl Siegel, one of the B.O.O.B.S. and "photo lady" extraordinaire, who along with photographer Jeff Gartin put our smiling faces on the back of the book as well as our individual portraits at the beginning of each story.

Many thanks to the staff of Cumberland House for all their hard work. Special gratitude to Ron Pitkin, who brought our vision to fruition with exceptional understanding and compassion. Lisa Taylor did a superb job designing and polishing the book. James Duncan's creative talents gave us an elegant and sensational cover.

Most of all, we wish to acknowledge the millions of women worldwide who are suffering from breast cancer. We stand together, connected not only by the common thread of our diagnosis, but also by our spirit to prevail until our enemy is vanquished.

B.O.O.B.S.

INTRODUCTION

My name is _____, and
I was diagnosed with breast cancer . . .

This was how we introduced ourselves at each meeting of our breast-cancer support group at The Wellness Community in Atlanta, Georgia. The first time, the words were hard to get out, but with each time it became easier. We were ten women for whom a normal day in our lives had suddenly become a living nightmare. We discovered that we were all asking the same questions:

- Why me? Did I do something to cause this?
- How much time do I have to live? Will I live?
- Should I seek a second, or even a third, opinion?
- Mastectomy or lumpectomy? How big will the scar be?
- Chemotherapy or radiation? Or both?
- Reconstruction or prosthesis? How will I look?
- What do mets, markers, and margins mean?
- I'm Stage 0; I'm Stage 4—should my stage be a concern?
- Should I take tamoxifen? Is it right for me?

We shared the same diagnosis, but we were a quilt of different patterns and colors. Our bodies and breasts came in an assortment of shapes, sizes, and shades. Our ages spanned twenty-five years. We came from various ethnic and economic backgrounds. Some of us were wives and mothers, grandmothers and great-grandmothers; some, single or divorced. Some of us were active in our careers; others, retired or no longer able to work. We had different religious beliefs. We had different occupations, lifestyles, and values. Even our breast cancer was diverse, varying from Stage 0 to Stage 4. We followed separate courses of surgeries and treatments.

We were not a bunch of statistics. We were not a female group of "genetic mishaps." We were—and still are—the voices of everyday, modern women struggling to survive breast cancer.

Despite our differences, we faced similar, overwhelming challenges, just to make it through each day. Life became complicated by our disease. In addition to our busy schedules and the physical aspects of our illness, we dealt with depression, work and disability issues, family and relationship crises, transportation problems, financial emergencies, and insurance hassles. We found ourselves enrolled in a crash course to learn and understand medical terminology and breast-cancer pathology.

We never had a clue how much stress our diagnosis would bring us. We were women others relied on, but despite our strength, many of the experiences were now too frightening, even for us.

In our support group, we felt safe enough to cry. Our scars and experiences connected us. We exchanged strategies for survival. We supported each other through the challenges we faced, whether surgery, chemotherapy, radiation therapy, or becoming "follically impaired." We formed an invincible bond.

We began to sense that a special purpose—beyond our disease—had brought us together. That purpose took shape in the form of a book—one that would give you, the reader, a front-row seat into the lives, minds, and bodies where breast cancer created both "visible" and "invisible" scars. We witnessed the transformation we each went through, and the inspiration and sisterhood that we experienced by having met one another.

We have discovered there is a new, heightened, and growing awareness of the disease and all its ramifications. Our mothers and grandmothers lived at a time when breast cancer was considered a social stigma and only discussed—whispered about—in private circles. Today, thanks to the efforts of various mainstream anti-cancer, educational, and fund-raising organizations, such as the American Cancer Society, National Cancer Institute, National Alliance of Breast Cancer Organizations, National Breast Cancer Coalition, and the Susan G. Komen Foundation, breast cancer has become a much more public and political issue in our country.

The rise of the feminist movement in the 1960s and '70s was instrumental in promoting breast-cancer activism, and a *new breed of survivors* began to emerge. One of the first women to challenge medical authority was Babette Rosmond, who offered her courageous viewpoint in her book, *The Invisible Worm*, in which she was critical of the Halsted radical mastectomy and wrote frankly of her decision not to have one. Rose Kushner, through her own breast cancer experience, wrote several landmark books. She was a pioneer in the crusade to allow women "access to complete and accurate health care information and the power to make their own decisions regarding their health." In 1979, a woman named Deena Metzger took a "warrior pose" against breast cancer when she allowed herself to be photographed, baring her mastectomy scar, which was covered with the tattoo of a tree. The world could no longer ignore what breast cancer *looked* like.

Betty Rollin, Betty Ford, Nancy Brinker, Fran Visco, and Susan Love, M.D. (to name a few) were at the forefront of new education, treatments, and many of the benefits breast-cancer patients now receive.

We have definitely come a long way, but despite the advances we've made, more than 210,000 American women will develop breast cancer this year, and about 40,000 American women will die of it. This number does not include the families, friends, and significant others whose lives are also, often traumatically, affected by this disease.

We ten women belong to this new breed of survivors. Our initiation began with our diagnosis, which took one of us into a "terrifying flight into the unknown." Another thought she was "bulletproof," another "wished the tumor would go away," another experienced "the most profound changes that had ever occurred in her life," another had an endless "long bald summer." Cancer intruded into all of our lives at untimely occasions—birthdays, holidays, weddings, anniversaries, putting on hold our many hopes, plans, and dreams for the future.

When one of the women in this book declared herself not *dying* of cancer, but *living* with it, her "take" on the disease gave us new insight, and even humor, in order to better cope.

As cancer transfigured our bodies, so it transformed our lives. We became resilient, resourceful, and, armed with information from the Internet, we were more informed than women had ever been. We explored our options and frequently combined alternative therapies in our recovery. A new sense of spirituality healed many of our emotional wounds. We learned to go within, to reprioritize what was important in our lives, to appreciate "being in the moment," and to find the peace and serenity that lies at the core of every human being.

We began to spread our wings—speaking to special interest groups and ethnic group gatherings, mentoring newly-diagnosed patients, becoming patient advocates, helping to raise money for breast-cancer organizations, and becoming board members of survivor support groups. We were too *busy* to die. Instead, we chose to help redefine the future for women—one without breast cancer.

Our silhouettes may have been altered, but not our spirits. We offer our stories to enlighten, encourage, and empower those of you who are about to get to know the Bunch Of Outrageous Breast-cancer Survivors, also known as the B.O.O.B.S.

Beverly Flowers

*has been a flight attendant with
American Airlines for nearly thirty
years. She was born in south Georgia,
but spent her childhood in
Connecticut. She attended Spelman
College in Atlanta where she earned a
bachelor's degree in early childhood
education. Married for seven years,
Beverly and her husband met in
church. Along with a strong faith,
Beverly feels blessed to have a close-
knit family and looks forward to seeing them often in spite of the fact that
they live all over the country. In her
free time she enjoys shopping and antiquing with friends, and to stay
in shape, she skis and rollerblades. She is very involved as a cancer
patient advocate for Northside Hospital through programs such as the
Network of Hope and The Wellness Community.*

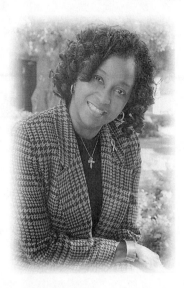

DIAGNOSIS PROFILE

Age at diagnosis:	45 years old
Family history:	None
Symptoms:	None—abnormal mammogram
Surgery:	Needle biopsy
	Mastectomy
	TRAM flap reconstruction
Biopsy results:	Infiltrating ductal carcinoma
	Stage: 1
	Tumor size: 1.5 cm.
	Nodes: 15 negative
	Grade: 1
	Estrogen receptor positive
	HER2/neu positive
Chemotherapy:	Adriamycin/Cytoxan (AC)
Hormonal therapy:	Tamoxifen

If breast cancer struck only men, there would be a cure.

Flight into the Unknown—
Destination: Breast Cancer

BEVERLY FLOWERS

Tuesday, September 11, 2001, appeared to be just an ordinary day—familiar, normal, and unexceptional. For many, it was the beginning of the countdown to the weekend, but I had important plans and a full agenda for that day.

Recently, I had celebrated my twenty-fifth anniversary as an American Airlines flight attendant. On Tuesday morning, I was rushing to the airport to make a 9:50 a.m. departure from Atlanta to St. Louis for a training session that would equip me to save the lives of passengers or fellow crew members on my flights. I was going to be trained and certified on the Automatic External Defibrillator (AED), a device that has been used successfully to save the lives of many passengers who had experienced sudden cardiac arrest. When operated correctly, the AED analyzes heart rhythms and, if necessary, delivers electrical shocks directly to the heart. The procedure brings to mind scenes from the hit TV show *E.R.*, when the doctor yells at the top of his lungs, "All clear!" before he delivers cardiac shocks to the patient's bare chest.

I was excited about receiving AED training because it would prepare me to be a guardian angel at 35,000 feet. It would also give prospective passengers a further sense of well-being and security about flying, because they would know that if they experienced a heart attack or heart failure, flight attendants could not only administer CPR (as we have done for years) but were also now qualified to use the AED.

Tuesday, September 11th, I entered the FAA restricted area to the American Airlines operations office at 8:46 a.m. And then, the unthinkable, the incomprehensible, happened. I suddenly heard screaming and running. I turned to walk down the corridor as one of my coworkers, an airline ticket agent, was running through the hallway. With a look of horror on her face, she cried out, "An airplane has just crashed into one of the twin towers of the World Trade Center in New York City!"

I was startled, perplexed, in a state of confusion. I was having trouble processing this information. Just moments earlier, I was contemplating how many lives I might save with my knowledge and operation of the AED, and now. . . . Was this some sort of terrible mistake or sick joke? My mind raced as I tried to figure out what was really going on. My very first thought was that a small, private aircraft, such as a Cessna, had hit the skyscraper.

I rushed to the nearest phone and called my husband, Roland, at our home. To my utter horror, shock, and dismay, not only did he confirm that an American Airlines plane had, in fact, crashed into the South Tower of the World Trade Center, he also said that he had just witnessed, "live" on television, a second plane crash into the North Tower. And that both towers were burning out of control! Then came the news of the Pentagon plane crash and the fourth plane that blew up in a Pennsylvania field, and it was all too obvious that these disasters were part of a well-organized terrorist plot on American soil, involving four United States commercial aircraft.

As soon as I had finished talking to Roland, the disbelief and sickening horror of what had happened began to sink in, and I became numb and weak, devoid of all strength and power. I felt totally helpless. I could feel the warmth, physically and emotionally, draining from my body. I was figuratively and literally cold—ice cold. Fear of the unknown began to slowly creep in and permeate my entire being. I sat down and my mind took flight to another time, another place, another day when I had that same numb feeling, that feeling of being devoid of all strength and power, the feeling of total defeat, the feeling of being cold—ice cold. And then, it dawned on me. It had been exactly two years ago: September 11th, at almost the exact same time of the morning. That was the day I was diagnosed with breast cancer!

*　*　*　*

Flashback. It was time for me to have my annual gynecological checkup, so I made an appointment to see my doctor. Following his examination, which included a Pap test, breast exam, cholesterol, blood pressure, and heart rate, he asked me to make an appointment for my mammogram. There was no urgency, so I waited a couple of weeks to set up the appointment. Since last year's results were fine, I considered it to be just another routine exam.

Roland and I left for the hospital, and as we drove I began complaining about not looking forward to having my breast smashed flat as a pancake. He said he did not even want to imagine how painful it must be. But I also said it was worth a little discomfort to make sure I was healthy.

The radiologist at South Fulton Medical Center in Atlanta, Georgia, who did the mammogram informed me that the results would be sent to my gynecologist within three days, and he would notify me if there were any problems. I was quite certain that everything was going to be fine. I returned home to what I considered "life as usual." Roland and I had been married for three years at the time and were still enjoying the title of "newlyweds." We would take our daily morning walks around our neighborhood, spotting deer in the woods across the street from our home. I enjoyed cooking chicken and vegetable stir-fry for him and making his favorite dish, saffron rice and fried plantains.

Naturally, as a flight attendant, I am away from home a couple of days a week, so the time spent with my husband and family is particularly pleasurable. I take none of them for granted.

The following week, I received a message on our voice-mail to call my gynecologist. I still did not have any reason to believe something was seriously wrong. I knew I had a history of high cholesterol and figured the doctor wanted to put me on cholesterol-lowering drugs. When I finally was able to speak directly to my gynecologist, he said, "Mrs. Flowers, we need to have you come into the office to discuss your mammogram and, if possible, you need to bring your husband with you." My heart sank. I asked myself what this could be. A few days later, Roland and I were sitting across the desk from my gynecologist in his office.

The first thing he said was, "We need the pictures from your last mammogram as soon as possible to compare the results." He continued after a second's pause. "There's an area in your left breast that needs to be examined by a surgeon." He asked me if I knew one. I told him I had only lived in Atlanta a short time, and because I had not had any medical problems I did not have a surgeon. He also asked me if I had experienced any lumps or pain in my left breast. My response was "no." I said I hadn't felt anything out of the ordinary. He recommended a biopsy and an ultrasound of my left breast, and asked to have the results sent to him as soon as possible.

Roland and I left the office not saying very much. Obviously something was wrong, but until we received the test results, we were certain this was just a little scare.

At this point, I was on a mission to find the best breast surgeon in the area. After making several phone calls to friends and family for recommendations, I finally decided on one from Breast Care Specialists.

I arrived at the doctor's office thirty minutes early. Roland had dropped me off. He was unable to stay with me because he had a prior business appointment. The friendly office staff put me at ease, and after a brief visit with the doctor, we proceeded with the needle biopsy.

The procedure wasn't painful, just a bit uncomfortable in the area where the needle was inserted. The doctor reassured me that she would call me at home with the results as soon as they were returned from the pathologist. I returned home, feeling relieved, knowing the biopsy was over, and now all I had to do was wait for the results. Several days passed, and I still had not heard from the doctor.

On September 11th, I left home for the airport to work my usual trip from Atlanta to St. Louis, Missouri. I arrived at Hartsfield-Jackson International Airport around 9:00 a.m. As I waited in the flight attendants' lounge before boarding my flight, I was told I had a phone call. I couldn't imagine who could be calling me at work, but I rushed into the office and picked up the phone. It was Roland, telling me that my doctor had called to speak to me about the results of the needle biopsy. I immediately phoned the doctor's office. I was put on hold and my anxiety escalated. By the time the receptionist returned to the phone and said, "The doctor will be right with you," my heart was beating so hard I felt as if it were trying to leap out of my chest.

"Good morning, Mrs. Flowers," were the next words I heard. "And how are you?" the doctor asked.

"I'm fine," I replied.

Then she asked, "Where are you?" I told her I was at the airport about to leave town for my trip to St. Louis and I would be returning later that evening. She said she had the results of the needle biopsy and that she could either tell me now or I could come in tomorrow and set up an appointment for my ultrasound. I said, "Please, tell me now. I'm sure I'll be okay."

There was a short pause and then I heard, "Beverly, I'm so sorry to have to tell you that you have breast cancer." I went numb. I didn't cry or say anything. The doctor went on to say that she would make the appointment for an ultrasound. It would pinpoint the exact location of the cancer. Ultrasound also determines if a lump is solid, a fluid-filled cyst, or a cancerous mass. A gel is placed on the surface of the breast to make it slippery, and a transducer is moved over the breast, sending waves through it to determine the characteristics of a lump. The procedure would be done the following week.

I hung up the phone and just stood there, thinking *this cannot be happening to me. There must be some mistake.* I didn't have any problems with my breasts, nothing that would concern me or make me think that I could possibly have breast cancer.

Why me? I had absolutely no family history of the disease. None of the women in my immediate family had any breast problems of any kind. I had always thought that women diagnosed with breast cancer were older and had a family history of breast cancer. Not only did I think breast cancer struck women only, I also thought it struck women who had neglected their health. Based upon my limited knowledge, I assumed that the majority of women diagnosed with breast cancer were heavy drinkers and/or smokers. I never smoked or drank heavily. *So why me?* I assumed that the majority of women diagnosed with breast cancer were significantly overweight. I'm 5′9″ and weigh 145 pounds. *So why me?* I assumed that women with breast cancer consumed large quantities of red meat and other high-fat foods. I rarely eat red meat—my diet consists mainly of chicken, seafood, turkey, and a variety of fruits and vegetables. *So why me?* I assumed that women with cancer were sedentary and out of shape. I have always been physically fit, and I love the outdoors. I ski and rollerblade. I am a lifetime, active health club member, and I work out regularly. *So why me?* I assumed that women with breast cancer were not informed and did not do monthly breast self-examinations or have yearly mammograms. Religiously every month, I did the self-exams, always checking, looking and feeling for lumps, discoloration, discharges, or other physical changes, and was always grateful when I did not find anything unusual. *So why me?* I further assumed that women with breast cancer were plagued with tremendous stress or emotional instability. My life was as stress-free as realistically possible in today's society. *So why me?*

*   *   *   *   *

My career as a flight attendant began in 1975. My first flight was from JFK International Airport, nonstop to London's Heathrow Airport. I boarded the Boeing 747 with excitement and anticipation. Many of the flight attendants working this flight had been flying for ten years or more, very senior. Being at the bottom of the seniority list, I realized that I would be awarded the last and least desirable position on this flight: E-Zone—the smoking section. Although a nonsmoker, as the most junior flight attendant, I had no choice.

After takeoff, the no-smoking and seat-belt signs were turned off simultaneously. Our approximate flying time to London was six and a half hours. I began to set up the galley located in the rear of the aircraft. The passengers appeared anxious to have their cocktails and dinner as soon as possible. After setting up the beverage cart, I was overwhelmed by the odor of cigarette smoke. My assigned section seated approximately fifty-two smoking passengers. The smoke was so thick in this area that it looked like an early morning fog. I could not see beyond five rows in front of me!

Smoking was allowed in this section for the duration of the flight, from shortly after takeoff to just prior to landing. I watched fifty-two smokers sit with cigarette in hand, eyes glued to the no-smoking sign, impatiently waiting for that moment when they could simultaneously "start their engines." I was subjected to fifty-two people chain-smoking cigarettes for six and a half to eight hours, two to three days per week, for ten consecutive years. Still, I felt somewhat impervious to the consequences of smoking because, after all, I did not smoke. Although my hair, skin, and uniform reeked of cigarette smoke after every flight, I always thought of it as an inconvenience rather than a detriment to my health. In the '70s and early '80s, little factual information was available on the dangers and consequences of secondhand smoke.

Today, it has been proven that secondhand smoke is not only harmful to our lungs, but is also known to cause certain types of cancer. I cannot prove that working for ten years in this smoke-filled environment caused my breast cancer, but I do believe in my heart that it was a contributing factor.

* * * * *

After the doctor's phone call, I walked out of the flight attendants' lounge and upstairs onto the airplane. I did not mention a word of my illness to my coworkers. I was still in shock. I could not bring myself to tell anyone that I had just, moments earlier, been diagnosed with a life-threatening illness—not even my husband. I was trying to push the words *breast cancer* back into the far corners of my mind so that I could perform my duties as a flight attendant—just as I had done for the past twenty-plus years. As I stood at the door of the MD-80 aircraft, I greeted each passenger with a friendly hello and a big smile. I was smiling on the outside but crumbling on the inside. The fear of the unknown and having so many unanswered questions about breast cancer—*my breast cancer*—were almost unbearable. I just could not, or did not, want to believe this was happening to me. When I returned home from my trip that evening, the first thing Roland asked was, "What did the doctor say to you today?"

"She needs to do an ultrasound, and I have to see her tomorrow," I replied. Denial and disbelief still consumed me. And, of all times for this to be happening to me. Roland and I had recently discussed trying to start a family. I was certain this would put that idea on hold for a while, and at forty-five years of age, my biological clock was ticking!

I arrived at the doctor's office around noon the next day, and as I was waiting in the reception area, I noticed a man seated with a large, brown envelope at his side. My first thought was that his wife or "significant other" was in the restroom and he was holding her envelope. Or could it be he's here for a breast exam too? I knew that a tiny percentage of breast-cancer patients are men, but still, he seemed somewhat out of place. When my name was called, I was ushered into the examination room where I patiently waited for the doctor's arrival. Upon entering the room, she immediately put me at ease. She was so pleasant and her demeanor was one of genuine concern for my well-being.

Following the ultrasound procedure, which took about ten minutes, the nurse told me to get dressed, that the doctor would return in a few minutes with the results. When the doctor finally returned, she took my hand in hers and looked at me compassionately. Before she said a word, I had hoped that, perhaps, she was going to say, "Beverly, you won't believe this, but the earlier results were misread. There was a terrible mix-up and you're just fine." Of course, deep down inside, I knew that would not be the case.

The doctor's first words to me were, "How are you feeling, Beverly?" I told her I felt fine. But of course, I was falling apart on the inside. She had my test results from the ultrasound. There were two cancerous lesions in my left breast positioned in two different locations, nine o'clock and twelve o'clock.

"What do we do now?" I asked. At that moment, all I wanted to know was how do I remove this cancer—this alien, this enemy, this evil, this sickness—from my body and from my life forever. I wanted to scream at the top of my lungs, *Cancer get out, go away, leave me and my family alone! This is not fair. What did I do to deserve this?* I wanted someone to shake me and wake me up from this terrible nightmare.

I paged Roland and told him he needed to come to the doctor's office, where I would be waiting for him. In the meantime, I had to prepare myself to tell him something that I knew would change both our lives. When Roland arrived at the office, I saw him through the plate-glass window, walking swiftly, and I could see the look of concern in his eyes. He sat down next to me—I was alone in the receptionist area.

"What did the doctor say about the biopsy?" he asked immediately.

I looked into his eyes. My voice was calm. "I have breast cancer, Roland." I had only seen tears in his eyes once before—at our wedding.

"Beverly, you know I lost my mom to cancer," Roland said. "And I don't want to lose you." Tears were streaming down his cheeks.

Sitting across from my doctor, I began to fire questions at her about my diagnosis. What kind of surgery did I need? Did I need to have a lumpectomy, a procedure that involves removing the lump from the breast, followed by radiation treatments? Or did I require a total mastectomy, the removal of the entire breast and surrounding tissue? And, if this was the case, would I have reconstruction? Had the cancer spread to my other breast or other parts of my body? How advanced or how fast was this cancer growing? Was the cancer found in time? Was I going to die?

Thus began my journey into the unknown.

We discussed my surgical options. The doctor explained to me that because I had cancer in two separate areas of my breast, she recommended a mastectomy instead of a lumpectomy, followed by reconstruction. Cosmetically, the lumpectomy would create two separate indentations on the surface of my breast that would not be very attractive. So, the mastectomy was what I chose.

I finally made the choice to have breast reconstruction after a lot of soul-searching and prayer. I knew that I would have a difficult time seeing myself without my breast. After my doctor told me that I would "come to the hospital with a breast and leave with a breast," I knew I had made the right decision.

My doctor referred me to a plastic surgeon who was also highly recommended by a close friend who had had reconstructive surgery following a mastectomy and was very happy with the results. Roland went with me for the initial consultation, and after that whenever possible, he was at my side.

I was very impressed by the plastic surgeon's genuine desire to make sure I was informed and felt comfortable about having reconstruction. He described the procedure called the TRAM flap. He told us that in order to create the new breast, he would use excess abdominal tissue to rebuild the breast mound. The operation would be performed immediately following the mastectomy and would require three to five days in the hospital. He also told me I would spend four to six weeks at home recovering and that I would have to use extreme caution when lifting or pulling objects during this time. But he reassured me that, in about six months, I could return to a normal routine.

I recommend to any woman who has had a mastectomy or is considering one that she learn as much as possible about breast cancer and breast reconstruction. Search the Internet and explore resources at the local library. Then find the best plastic surgeon in the area. Having reconstruction following a mastectomy can definitely improve a woman's self-confidence and body image. For me, it was a tremendous boost to my self-esteem and general well-being—mentally and physically. I would definitely do it again if I had to. And, like my close friend, I, too, am very pleased with the results. My breasts are normal now, and there were no complications from the surgery. I have been truly blessed.

But I wondered at times if I should feel guilty about having had the reconstructive surgery. I vividly remember watching a PBS documentary many years ago in which a woman who had undergone a bilateral mastectomy chose not to have reconstruction. This cancer survivor also chose not to wear any type of breast prosthesis. She said that she was comfortable with her body and her husband still found her desirable. Even back then, as I watched the documentary, I remember thinking that I would not be comfortable having a mastectomy without reconstruction. *Vanity, vanity, vanity,* I guess.

Still, I had this momentary guilt about wanting to see two perfectly normal-looking breasts when I showered. Two perfect breasts when I dressed or undressed in front of a mirror. Two perfect breasts when I was with my husband during our intimate moments. Two perfect breasts when I undressed in front of other women at the local gym. And, of course, two perfect breasts when I wore my favorite bathing suit.

Despite this brief period of guilt—the operative word being *brief*—I am definitely an "overcomer" and true survivor. Through prayer, education, and wisdom I came to a revelation that brought me both peace and understanding. I realized that I am an individual; I am unique. I am thankful I did not make the same decision the woman in the documentary made. I respect and applaud her decision. She did what she felt was right for her. And I did what was necessary and right for me.

Breasts. Two things that made Marilyn Monroe, and so many other women like her, sex symbols. Breasts that secrete milk to nourish babies. Breasts that lovers admire, fondle, caress. Breast enlargements, breast reductions, breast implants; here a breast, there a breast, everywhere a breast! Large ones, small ones, round ones, even short ones and long ones! Boobs everywhere! *But when cancer invades them, they take on a whole new, frightening image.*

I continued to work, and tried to maintain my daily routines as if everything were okay. I refused to allow myself to fall into a well of despair and self-pity. I knew in my heart that I had a long journey through unknown territory—breast cancer was attacking my body. I was determined to do everything I could to return to the lifestyle I had before breast cancer invaded my life.

It was now one week before Thanksgiving and, of course, the Christmas holidays were fast approaching. How was I going to prepare myself and my family for what was going to happen to me within the next several months?

On Thanksgiving, I truly felt thankful that I was headed to a joyous gathering consisting of my family, which included my husband, my mother (my dad had passed away eleven years earlier), my dearest and only brother, Reginald, sister-in-law, Elaine, and darling nieces, Melanie and Blayre.

This was not a dreaded, obligatory holiday gathering. I am always overjoyed to be in the company of my small but close-knit family. Why, then, was I filled with such overwhelming trepidation at the thought of this particular trip at this festive time of the year? I knew my mother would be busy in the kitchen preparing a traditional southern Thanksgiving dinner with all the trimmings. The golden-brown turkey, succulent cornbread dressing, freshly picked collard greens, yellow squash, candied yams, cranberry sauce and, of course, the homemade sweet potato pies, and the always delicious sour cream and butter pound cake.

As Roland and I waited at the airport for our flight to Dallas on that Thanksgiving morning, I turned and noticed my husband looking at me with deep love and tremendous concern. I knew that I should be feeling eternally grateful for all my blessings, but I found myself emotionally sinking on the inside, and working very hard to maintain a sense of bravado on the outside. As we boarded the plane, I realized this was the first time in my life that I really did not want to face my beloved mother, the woman who had always been my trusted friend, constant companion, mentor, and spiritual counselor.

As Roland and I fastened our seat belts for takeoff, I asked God to give me the strength to face my mom with integrity and solicit her love, support, and wisdom in the coming battle. The Delta L-1011, with its three powerful engines, drowned out many sounds as we taxied down the runway, but it could not drown out the sound of two words that were blasting in my head—*breast cancer!*

When we finally arrived in Dallas, the sinking feeling I had in the pit of my stomach actually made it hard for me to walk. In about one hour, my family would know I was diagnosed with breast cancer, and truthfully, I wasn't sure I would live long enough to celebrate the Christmas holidays with them!

After the wonderful Thanksgiving dinner, I asked my mother if I could talk to her privately. We went upstairs to her room. I nestled comfortably on the bed and said as simply as I could, "Mom, I have breast cancer." I was not sure how she was going to react. To my surprise, she was very calm and told me that she would be with me through it all. My mother has a strong faith in God, and I knew her prayers would be answered. In her mind, recovery was certain. Telling the rest of my family about my diagnosis was not as difficult as I had anticipated, and our short stay in Plano was quite enjoyable, after all.

Roland and I returned to Atlanta and began preparing our home for the Christmas holiday. I only had about two weeks before surgery. We went Christmas shopping—I didn't want my recovery period to interfere with buying and wrapping presents—and we were still expecting my brother and his family to visit us in Atlanta during the holidays. Roland and I purchased a seven-foot, majestic Canadian fir tree and spent several days decorating it with beautiful ornaments and carefully arranging all the gifts under it. I was determined that breast cancer would not alter my lifestyle. Christmas holiday preparations helped me to cope with the uneasy feelings I had about my impending surgery.

In December, Roland and I arrived at Northside Hospital for my preoperative appointment. When we returned home, my mother was there to accompany us to the hospital the following morning. The time had finally arrived for me to begin my journey. As they were about to wheel me into the operating room, Mom reassured me that with God and her prayers she knew I would be okay. Roland, his eyes filled with love and a hint of fear, accompanied me to the pre-op area, where he kissed me and told me he loved me. I told him that I was going to win this battle and not to worry.

My husband, like so many men, was taught to be the strong one in the face of danger and the unknown. Unfortunately, Roland knew something about both, and he did not like what he knew. He was born in Panama and raised in New York City by a loving, independent, single mother who was a nurse by profession. As an only child, Roland and his mother had an extremely close bond. After telling Roland that she had been diagnosed with cancer, her health deteriorated quickly and she was forced to stop working as a pediatric nurse, a position she truly loved and enjoyed. Roland took a leave of absence from his job to care for and support her through this crisis. Three months later, his beloved mother succumbed to cancer. When I received my diagnosis, I knew Roland would be very upset. I also knew he would be in my corner for the biggest fight of my life.

The stakes were high; I was literally in a fight *for* my life. I said to my opponent, breast cancer, "You have picked the wrong person to step into the ring with. You may win a couple of rounds, but I will win this fight!"

No one wants to face a powerful enemy alone. As I looked in my corner, I realized it was, in fact, overcrowded with help and support and love. First of all there was God, then my husband, my mother, the spirit of my late beloved father, my brother, my sister-in-law, my wonderful nieces, my aunts, my cousins, and my close friends. My medical support team served their fighter admirably, from the Georgia Cancer Specialists group to the Atlanta Plastic Surgery group, to the Breast Care Specialists group. Every corner also has a trainer—I had the Northside Hospital Occupational Therapist group. With this type of support, I was not going to lose this fight!

My mastectomy and reconstructive surgery were a success. Losing my breast was a small price to pay, considering this procedure would probably save my life. Believe me, it was a frightening thought not knowing whether this treatment would make me cancer-free. At this time, I still did not have the results of my pathology report, which would tell me whether or not the cancer was contained; that is, just in the left breast.

When I finally woke up after several hours in recovery, I was brought back to my room, a bit groggy but awake, thank God. I had so much to be thankful for and was pleased to see my mom, husband, and cousins Stan and Cheryl waiting there for me.

I was a bit sore near my breast area, but overall, the pain was minimal. The nursing staff at Northside Hospital, in charge of my care, was fantastic. They showed great concern for my well-being and recovery. The second day after surgery, the nurses made sure I was up, out of bed, and taking short walks. My doctors were there to check my progress, daily. I knew I still had a long journey ahead of me—I wanted my life back.

Now, I was preparing myself for the day when I would actually see my new breast for the first time. Of course you visualize what you may look like, but I felt confident that I would be pleased with the results.

I was home, after three days in the hospital, sitting on my bed and looking inside my gown to see my reconstructed breast. I touched it gently. It felt a little firmer than my natural breast. My husband assured me that the breast looked beautiful and I still had cleavage.

Having reconstructive surgery was right for me. I knew when I walked into the hospital for surgery that I would leave with both my breasts. I also knew how pleased I would be to have a flat stomach! The fatty tissue from the "tummy tuck" is used to create the new breast. So, even though I had had two major surgeries that December, I would not have wanted to do it any other way.

It felt so good to come home. It really felt good to smell the fresh air and see other people going about their daily lives, walking, driving, shopping, going to movies and restaurants. Soon I would be up and about again, and back to normal. But what I still did not know at this time was if the cancer had spread. My doctor assured me that as soon as she received my pathology report, she would telephone with the results. Needless to say, every time the phone rang, my heart would start pounding. However, I was emotionally prepared to handle the results even if they were not favorable. The doctor called three days later to tell me that she received my pathology report and she had great news. "We examined fifteen of your lymph nodes, and none were involved," she said. This meant the cancer had not spread to any other part of my body. It was the best news I could have received. For the first time, I knew I was about halfway through the journey with cancer.

In the days following my surgery, I tried, as best I could, to return to a "normal" life. My mom had moved into our home temporarily to care for me; she cooked delicious meals. She also accompanied Roland and me to all my checkups and ran errands, especially to the local pharmacy for my medical needs. And above all, my mother's love and faith in God was forever present during my illness. She prayed with me and for me every single day.

I was determined to make this Christmas holiday the best one ever, despite my cancer. On Christmas Day, I put on makeup and my favorite blouse, and Mom combed my hair. As I opened presents and sang Christmas carols with my family, I felt relatively happy, though I knew that soon I'd have to take another journey into unknown territory—chemotherapy.

Following my initial consultation with Dr. G. of Georgia Cancer Specialists, I found myself facing the greatest challenge of my life. The doctor explained, with my mother and Roland present, what chemotherapy was all about. I was overwhelmed with information. For the first time, I began reconsidering my decision to go through the treatment at all! I had seen and heard so many horror stories about the side effects of chemotherapy. Hair loss, weight loss, vomiting, and nausea—I was not ready to deal with any of these changes. As a patient, it was so difficult to believe that these powerful drugs, and all their side effects, were actually going to *help* me. I did not want to hear that I had to be sick again in order to be well again.

Although my prognosis was good, my chances for recurrence were greater if I did not have chemotherapy. This dilemma took its toll on me emotionally. In fact, my mental state was the lowest it had been since my cancer diagnosis. I lost my appetite and began having feelings of hopelessness, which were driving me into a deep depression. I also became resigned to the chemo course of treatment. I had been convinced that any other alternative was not a smart option. And doing nothing would really be a foolish choice.

The following week, I was scheduled for my first of four cycles of chemotherapy. As we drove to the Georgia Cancer Specialists office, I found it very hard to concentrate on anything other than the day of my final treatment. My twenty-one-day cycle meant that I would come to the office for an injection every three weeks. The drugs were administered intravenously, and the treatment sessions usually lasted about two hours.

Actually, my first visit went quite well. The only problem was when my oncology nurse had a hard time finding a vein to insert the IV into. The chemotherapy room had about twenty lounge chairs, and I was happily surprised to see other patients who appeared to be coping quite well. Some were talking and joking with the nursing staff and munching on snacks. Seeing this eased my anxiety, and helped me to realize that I could overcome my fears of chemotherapy.

The anti-nausea medication I was given made me a bit sleepy, and I was a little tired the next day, but not as bad as I had anticipated. Mom and I were able to go out and do some shopping, which is one of my favorite pastimes and, therefore, made me feel that I wasn't putting my life on hold.

The following week, I returned to the doctor's office for my blood work. Unfortunately, the results were not what I expected. I was told that my white blood cell count was at a level too low to continue with the chemotherapy treatments. Dr. G. informed me that I would need to have Neupogen injections—a drug designed to return my white blood cell count to an acceptable level. This delay in treatment was very disappointing, even though the doctor assured me that it's a common occurrence. I returned to the doctor's office every day for a week to receive an injection. Then, I asked the oncology nurse if it were possible for me to administer my own injections. She said yes, and showed me how to do it. I was so glad to be able to do it, not only to save myself the one-hour drive to the office but also because I felt more comfortable administering my own injection.

The Neupogen appeared to work, although it caused severe bone pain. Finally, the blood count increased and I was able to begin my second cycle of chemotherapy.

This was when I started to lose my hair. I would wake up in the morning and find large amounts of it on my pillow. Fortunately, my hair loss wasn't as traumatic as it might have been since I had prepared for it in advance by buying a wig that matched my natural hair color and style. Although I know that for some women the hair loss is traumatic, I believe the key to coping is to remember that it's a temporary side effect, and, after the last treatment, it begins to grow back. Sometimes, thicker or curlier, or even a different color!

It was definitely at this point in my treatment that extreme fatigue, both mental and physical, set in. I would now really need the help and support of close friends and family. My mother was also exhausted from spending so much time taking care of me. I was sure she needed a break, so my godparents, Bill and Fran Redman, drove down from Connecticut to help my mother. I was so fatigued that I spent most of my time either sitting in the bedroom or in bed, resting and reading.

During my third chemo treatment, Dr. G. said she was amazed at how well I was doing. I could not imagine why because I felt that I "looked sick," even though I still wore makeup as usual and dressed in my favorite outfits. Certain smells would trigger my nausea. I have to say that for me the weirdest side effect of chemotherapy was the temporary loss of my normal sense of taste and smell. My favorite perfume smelled like rubbing alcohol! The very smell of food cooking reminded me of the local landfill.

Dr. G. informed me during one visit that she hoped I would be interested in participating in a television segment on coping with chemotherapy (for women with breast cancer). She explained that other women would see me as an example of someone who, although I had surgery and chemotherapy, was able to overcome the disease that had unexpectedly invaded my life.

In January, I received a call from the health reporter at Fox 5, the local Atlanta affiliate of Fox Television. The segment was filmed in my home. One of the first things I said on camera was that breast cancer is not a death sentence. In fact, early detection is a woman's greatest defense against this dreaded disease. I conveyed the good news that life can and will return to normal if you keep a positive attitude. I wanted to reach out to other women with breast cancer to show them that no matter how long the journey, they can make it. The most important thing was to never give up hope.

At last, my final chemotherapy treatment. It was something I had looked forward to for a long time. I said my goodbyes to the office staff with whom I had developed a special bond. They had been there to answer any questions and to hold my hand, if needed. So, as much of a bumpy ride as chemotherapy was, I could now look forward to "smoother air."

Following my chemo treatments, slowly but surely, my energy returned. My surgeon recommended I begin sessions with an occupational therapist to help me regain full motion of my left arm, and for strength training to prepare me for my return to work. I met with the occupational therapist at Northside Hospital twice a week. She put me through such an intense workout that it brought me to tears the first two weeks. I had an intense dislike for her "methods of pain," but I loved her for pushing me to my physical limits. When I began physical therapy, I was lifting two-pound weights. After five months, I was lifting fifty pounds! I also continued to walk daily. My main concern at this point was to prepare myself not only physically, but mentally, to return to work.

During one of my numerous trips back to Northside Hospital, I was approached in A Woman's Place (the boutique in the lobby of the Women's Center that specializes in clothing, gifts, and books for women with breast cancer) by Barbara Robey, a social worker. She recognized me from the Fox 5 television segment, in which she had also appeared. We went to Starbucks together and discussed the TV show, and then Barbara asked me if I would be interested in joining a breast-cancer support group. I was not sure if I was ready to participate or become involved, but Barbara was very convincing and we set up an interview for me to join a pilot group of breast-cancer survivors—The Network of Hope.

After my interview, I was chosen as one of the original breast-cancer survivors whose responsibilities included calling newly diagnosed breast-cancer patients at home following surgery to address any concerns, fears, or problems they may encounter during their treatment and recovery.

This select group of women have become a second family to me. We have monthly meetings where we gather to have a light dinner, talk, laugh . . . and sometimes cry. Susan Lucier, the breast-cancer coordinator at Northside Hospital, has put her heart and soul into making our group a successful tool for all the breast-cancer patients admitted to Northside. This group has changed my life forever. We are definitely "sisters with a cause." Our monthly meetings, held at The Wellness Community, have been the best support system anyone could hope for. The Wellness Community, along with its outstanding classes and seminars, provides a wealth of information, not only for breast-cancer survivors, but also for other types of cancer survivors, as well as support for survivors' family members.

* * * * *

In October 2000, Breast Cancer Awareness Month, I attended my first "Walk for the Cure," with other members of the Network of Hope. My eyes filled with tears when I first saw the thousands of pink hats and T-shirts worn by survivors as we participated in our annual walk. It gave me renewed hope that someday soon there will be a cure for breast cancer.

My return to work after nine months was rather uneventful. I walked onto the plane knowing that my breast-cancer journey had ended, and that I was once again headed for a familiar destination: St. Louis, Missouri.

I have continued my work with the Network of Hope, and I recently began hospital visits to newly diagnosed breast-cancer patients. I present, as a gift, a Susan G. Komen bear, a stress-free ball, a small comfort pillow, and a personalized letter from the Northside Hospital Auxiliary. These hospital visits were difficult for me at first—when I would see a patient in bed, I would look at her and see myself. But after visiting several women, it became much easier for me. I *wanted* to give them hope and let them know that there is life after breast cancer. Of course, you emerge a different person, any life-threatening experience changes your perspective on life and reorganizes your priorities, but the greatest thing it does is to make you a stronger individual. I feel that after breast cancer I can handle any challenge life presents.

The song "I Will Survive" is now a powerful anthem for breast cancer. I found a whole new significance in its lyrics (which I had been singing since the 1970s) when viewed in the context of a breast-cancer survivor:

Did you think I would crumble
Did you think that I would just lay down and die!
Oh, no, not I, Oh no, not I
I will survive, I will survive.

*   *   *   *   *

In 2001, I was happily anticipating my twenty-fifth class reunion. I could hardly contain myself at the thought of seeing many of my former classmates from Spelman College, with whom I had graduated in May 1976. It was to be a weekend event with a formal cocktail party scheduled for Saturday night. I knew that what I wore to this party had to be the "perfect" outfit. It was difficult to decide, but I finally chose a tuxedo pantsuit with a silver and black bustier. This would be the first time since my surgery that I would dare to go braless and show cleavage!

I knew I had made the right decision when one of my classmates approached me and said, "Beverly, you look great tonight, and I love your bustier."

I politely replied, "Thank you."

Just before she turned to walk away, she said, "You still have those big, beautiful breasts."

She left me standing there with my mouth open, totally speechless. If she only knew that she was looking at my $30,000 breast! What a confidence-building moment that was, and one I will never forget. Once again, I could be proud of my physical image, and that went a long way in accelerating my healing process.

* * * * *

And so, September 11, 2001, before 8:46 a.m., was just an ordinary and unexceptional day. Then, in less than two hours our world changed forever. We would never be the same. We would certainly never feel safe in our own country again.

It was not easy to get back on a plane to do the job I loved and had been doing for the last twenty-seven years. Fear was now a constant traveling companion. Was my plane going to be the next one used as a weapon of mass destruction? I realized that I would have to prepare myself emotionally for every takeoff and landing. There were also the personal sadnesses: a coworker was now mourning the death of her brother, who was killed on the 91st floor of Tower One of the

World Trade Center. And a close college friend of mine lost his fiancée, who worked on the 101st floor of Tower Two.

The economic impact of 9/11 was also beginning to take its toll. Our flight attendant work force has been reduced by 20 percent, which led to many of my coworkers, some personal friends, being furloughed indefinitely. And this directly and adversely affected my work schedule. Service to certain cities has been reduced or totally eliminated, and the domino effect of that was a loss of jobs at airports, hotels, rental car agencies, and of course, travel agencies. Today, everyone I work with is concerned about being next on the furlough list—our sense of job security has been tragically taken from us. Right after 9/11, the airlines offered grief counseling services and leaves of absence due to stress. Many of my coworkers have yet to return to work; it has been too overwhelming for them. Ironically, I was already, emotionally and psychologically, in a survival mode as a result of my battle fought and won with breast cancer. I believe it gave me the mental fortitude to better deal with the events of 9/11.

But there are some changes and reminders that are hard to deal with. When the man known as "the shoe bomber" was caught, our crew of five and plane filled to capacity—140 passengers—was forced to remain on the tarmac for more than four hours as this breach of security unfolded. It was a terrifying reminder that we would never be safe. Of course, airport security has definitely been improved. Metal detection equipment has been upgraded. There are no curbside check-ins, and only two pieces of carry-on luggage per passenger are allowed. These days, sharp objects such as nail files, scissors, tweezers, even plastic eating utensils are confiscated. The National Guard is used at security checkpoints in addition to local law enforcement, and U.S. sky marshals now fly on selected flights. But as we are all well aware, no airport can be 100 percent secure at all times. Ironically, and not surprisingly, security has now taken on an unfortunate element: racial profiling by passengers. Anyone who appears to be of Arab or Middle Eastern descent is immediately subjected to stares of prejudice and mistrust. I'm sure this will go on for a long time.

One of the things I have learned to do, in order not to dwell on the tragedy, is to avoid watching documentaries about 9/11. I never again want to see the horrific sight of those planes crashing into the WTC and exploding. It only makes me relive that morning at Hartsfield-Jackson International Airport and remember the despair I felt upon realizing that thousands of people had died.

In March 2002, I flew to New York City for the first time since 9/11. As we were about to land, I looked out of the window at the Manhattan skyline and realized that the WTC buildings I had flown past hundreds of times were gone. A tremendous emptiness and an overwhelming sense of loss engulfed me. Over the years, whenever we flew to New York, the pilot would always point out over the PA two of New York's most famous landmarks: the Statue of Liberty and the World Trade Center. The pilot now says nothing.

The other strong feeling I am still left with is anger at the fact that terrorists were so easily able to dupe so many people: enroll in and successfully complete flight training school, obtain visas, and remain in this country unnoticed and unchallenged. I know it's a feeling that I share with millions of Americans. But as time goes by, my sense of dismay and defeat is being replaced by even stronger feelings of hope and victory.

Once again, I'm aware that every day of my life since that fateful September 11th when I was diagnosed with breast cancer has been a miraculous gift from God. Then, two years later on that same date, our country was attacked. The first taught me that I could face the fear and terror of my diagnosis and win. The latter was a day filled with a very different kind of terror, but one I think we Americans have the courage and strength to fight . . . and ultimately win.

❧

Beverly looks forward to finishing with tamoxifen in the coming year. She recently completed chemotherapy treatment for colon cancer and has resumed her active lifestyle. Her tremendous inner strength helps her maintain a positive outlook.

Beth Butler

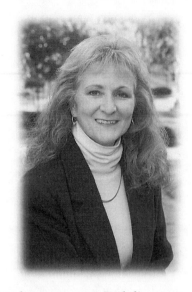

was born and raised in Augusta, Georgia. She has always been strong-willed, independent, and ambitious. Beth divorced young, and as a single mother she not only raised her own daughter from the age of four, but practically raised a niece as well. Focusing on her career in computer administration, she did well. Beth is an outdoor type, who likes snow skiing and camping, but most of all enjoys horseback riding. Magnum is her beloved horse and companion that she rescued almost twenty years ago, the same year she lost her mother to breast cancer. Beth lives on a sprawling farm, northeast of Atlanta, Georgia, with her four horses, three cats, and a dog.

DIAGNOSIS PROFILE

Age at diagnosis:	49 years old
Family history:	Mother, maternal aunt, maternal great-grandmother
Symptoms:	Self-discovered lump
Surgery:	Core biopsy
	Lumpectomy
	Axillary node dissection
Biopsy results:	Infiltrating ductal carcinoma
	Stage: 1
	Tumor size: 1.5 cm.
	Nodes: 11 negative
	Estrogen and progesterone receptors positive
	Grades: 1 & 2
	S phase: 12.6
	DNA: 1 of 2 types aggressive
Chemotherapy:	Cytoxan/methotrexate/5-FU (CMF)
Radiation therapy:	33 treatments
Hormonal therapy:	Tamoxifen

You don't get to choose how you're going to die.
Or when. You can decide how you're going to live now.

—Joan Baez

Five-Foot-Six
and Bulletproof

BETH BUTLER

Or at least I had always thought I was. I was forty-nine, single, with a grown daughter, and had what I considered a "good life." I had always, since early childhood, been healthy, active, independent, and ambitious. I divorced my husband in my late twenties, when I realized that both of us wanted such different things in life that we could never be happy if we stayed together. I dove into single motherhood and my professional life with a passion. I somehow managed to raise an absolutely wonderful daughter and, simultaneously, build a decent career in computer administration. It was always very important to me to be able to make it on my own before I could consider marriage again.

I have always loved outdoor sports, to the point that I have frequently been accused of having a death wish. If I couldn't get killed doing it, I wasn't interested. Over the years, I excelled at skiing, white-water rafting, horseback riding, parasailing, and just about anything else I had the chance to try. Along the way, there were several long-term relationships with good men, and one lasting, close friendship, but I never seriously considered marriage. There always seemed to be plenty of time for that . . . later. As I got a little older, I tended to date younger men because I found it hard to find anyone my own age who could keep up with me.

By the time I reached the ripe old age of forty-nine, I was living in my "dream house" (a farm, actually). My daughter, Alison, was out of college and happily married, living a five-hour drive away, and I was settled into a promising position as a software administrator with a large corporation. The farm, located in a small, rural town fifty miles north of Atlanta, had been a lifetime dream that I had worked toward with singular devotion. I am far enough from the city to be able to enjoy beautiful sunrises, sunsets, and bright, moonlit pastures where my horses graze. When my parents died, I used my inheritance to buy eight and a half acres of land and build the house and barn for me and my "boys" (three Tennessee Walkers that I love dearly). A dear friend, who somehow put up with me during the construction of the house and barn, helped me build a half-mile of wood fence and finish out the interior of the four-stall barn. It took a long time and was hard work, but I loved every minute.

I was involved in a relationship with Rick, a guy fourteen years my junior, who had shared my passion for horses and the outdoors. He owned the farm across the road, and our friendship quickly grew into a romantic relationship. He moved in with me after we had been seeing each other for about six months. We never really discussed the move, and I wasn't sure I was ready for it—I just allowed it to happen.

As long as I can remember, I have been "horse crazy." Growing up, I rode whenever I could and always dreamed of having my own horse. I think I must have asked Santa for a horse every Christmas of my childhood, but my parents would not even let me have a dog.

I'm not sure where my love of animals came from, but it definitely was not inherited. I finally bought my first horse when I was thirty-five years old. His name is Magnum, and he is now in his early twenties, and still with me. I bought him as a rescue from a guy I knew who was not taking care of him. I had ridden the horse and gotten along with him well, even though he was a bit high-strung. I named him Magnum because he was very big—and a real "pistol." We had our rough times learning from each other, but over the years we have become best friends. I think Magnum knows that no one else in the world would put up with him (or me!). Whenever I have had a particularly tough day, or just need to spend some time with my "inner self," I always head for the barn, even when I have boarded the horses. Magnum never seems to mind my presence, so I've spent many thoughtful (and tearful) hours brushing him or just sitting in a corner of his stall. My emotions run deep, and when put in highly emotional situations, I take my mind away from where I am by mentally brushing Magnum from head to tail. It has kept me from losing it at several funerals!

*   *   *   *   *

I lost my mother to breast cancer in 1985. My dad died of Alzheimer's in 1993. My maternal aunt was diagnosed with breast cancer in 1988 at the age of eighty-four and survived with only a mastectomy, but died of a stroke at the ripe old age of ninety-five. My maternal great-grandmother also died of breast cancer. This family history of cancer did not bode well for me. However, I always thought that I would be the one to get Alzheimer's because I was physically more like my father and his side of the family. His mother had also died of Alzheimer's. Having lost both parents to horrible diseases, I always said that if I had to die from one or the other, I would choose cancer any day! Those words would come back to haunt me.

My mother's battle with breast cancer began in 1979, when she was seventy-three years old. As was the common procedure at that time, they performed a radical mastectomy (negative nodes) with no follow-up treatment. I still do not know her exact diagnosis, but I do know that the tumor was very near the sternum. While the nodes were negative, her surgeon did not excise the nodes under the sternum (closest to the tumor) due to their location. Almost five years later, she had some pain in her lower back and hip, which turned out to be an inoperable malignancy on her spine. She went through the whole spectrum of radiation and chemo and finally lost her battle a year later. She was a real trooper through it all, and when she died, her mind was still clear and sharp. Both her daughters were at her side. Sadly, my father's Alzheimer's had progressed to the point where he never really knew she was gone. He lingered for eight more years.

Shortly after I had started construction on my farm, the division of the large electronics corporation that I worked for moved to another city. I was offered jobs in two different locations, but both would have meant relocating to places I didn't want to live, to say nothing of giving up the farm. I took a summer off to finish up the fence and barn, and during that time decided to take the plunge—I would start my own business. My expertise had always been in computers, but I also loved doing physical work and creating things with my hands. I followed in my sister and brother-in-law's footsteps and started a "design and build" closet/storage business. At the same time, I accepted a temporary, flexible-time position with a large corporation, working for a generous man who let me create my own schedule to allow time for the closet business. But between the two jobs, I ended up, rather predictably, working six or seven days a week, ten to twelve hours a day for about two and a half years. My business did not take off the way I had hoped, and the temporary job grew into a very challenging permanent job, shifting the closet business to a "nights and weekends" second job.

I was not as diligent about annual checkups and mammograms as I should have been. Remember, I was bulletproof. I had a baseline mammogram when I was thirty-eight or thirty-nine and repeat films done every two or three years. Not enough, given my family history. I had skipped a few years because I lacked good health insurance coverage, especially when I worked at the temporary job and was trying to build my own business. I intentionally did not have a mammogram during that time for fear that they would find something and that would create some financial hardship for me. Luckily, when I became a permanent, full-time employee with my present employer, I received excellent insurance coverage through the company.

At age forty-nine, in the late fall I noticed a small lump in my left breast. That sounds ominous as I write it, but it did not seem so at the time. I really did not think too much of it (why, I will never know!), but it did make me realize I was long overdue for a mammogram. I decided to schedule one, but getting the necessary insurance approvals and referrals became very difficult. The company was in the midst of changing insurance carriers, so I finally gave up and decided that I would have to wait until after the first of the year.

It took six weeks to get the mammogram scheduled. If I had been more insistent and told them I had found a lump, I am sure I could have gotten the appointment more quickly, but that was just another part of the denial. In mid-April I went alone for the mammogram. I told no one, not even Rick, and really was not nervous. I did tell the technician about the lump. She placed a little stick-on dot on my breast over the area to mark it. After the films were done, she had the radiologist review them before I left. The radiologist was the director of the Breast Center at the hospital, and she came out to tell me that she wanted to do an ultrasound that same day. She was a wonderful, caring doctor, who actually came in to see the ultrasound herself. She said that it looked like a benign, common type of tumor, but she wanted to do a "needle core biopsy" just to be sure. She repeatedly assured me not to worry. There was a five-day wait before the biopsy could be done because of an over-the-counter painkiller I had been taking for joint pain. I also had a three-day business trip planned during that time. The doctor again said it would be fine to wait until I returned. The appointment was made for April 23, the anniversary of my father's death.

At this point, I will admit that I went into the biopsy without learning anything else about the procedure other than what the doctor had told me. I have since learned how lucky I was to have the radiologist that I had. Several women I know have endured some pretty bad experiences with biopsies performed by doctors who made no effort to ease the pain and tension.

Again, I went alone, without telling anyone except Phil, my best friend of twenty years. He was the only one I trusted not to freak out. Besides, I did not want to worry my sister and daughter, or even Rick, in case it turned out to be only a benign cyst. Phil was visibly shaken but supportive. He said simply, "It's probably nothing, but whatever it is, we'll just deal with it."

The day of the biopsy, the nurse, technician, and doctor were all very compassionate and comforting. The director of the Breast Center, who had done the ultrasound, was also doing the biopsy. They dimmed the lights in the room and even brought in some soft music. The nurse held my hand while I watched the whole procedure on the monitor. They made sure I was comfortable and did everything possible to avoid pain. I found it interesting to watch the procedure on the monitor, and I still was not particularly concerned, although I was beginning to feel a bit apprehensive about the outcome. The results were due back in a few days, and I had asked them to please call me at work so that Rick would not accidentally get the message and ask questions I was not ready to answer. The doctor called late that afternoon and was very apologetic about originally having suggested that the lump was benign. Instead, it was malignant. I was facing breast cancer.

Pretty scary and unbelievable. Whatever happened to "bulletproof?" I somehow managed to not fall apart—I have a way of putting bad things aside to avoid panic. I finished up my day quickly and headed for home. I cried through most of the drive and when I got home, I phoned Phil and left him a message about the results. Then, I immediately changed clothes and went out to get Magnum. There was a thunderstorm brewing, but I did not really care. I saddled my best buddy and started out. Along the way, I passed Rick, who was repairing fence on his property. He tried to yell at me to go back because thunder and lightning were signaling the beginning of a typical southern storm. It was as though Mother Nature was responding to the turn my life had suddenly taken. Magnum and I went out to a nearby pasture and he cantered while I cried. He always knows when I am upset, and he took good care of me as we rode in the storm. Later that evening, I told Rick. He responded with a simple "I'm sorry." No hugs, no tears, just "I'm sorry."

I called my sister, Marian, that night and broke the news to her. I heard the fear in her voice as she said, "Oh, Beth, are you sure?" She and I had held each other up through our mother's and aunt's breast cancer. I knew those memories were flooding back to her, just as they were to me. I also told her that I wanted to wait until I found out about surgery before telling Alison.

In the morning I contacted my gynecologist to see what to do next. He referred me to a surgeon who offered to see me right away. In fact, I was asked if I could come in that same morning. That was when I began to understand the urgency of the situation. I scheduled an appointment for the following day to give me time to get the necessary insurance approvals. I felt a little uneasy about choosing a doctor without knowing anything about him. When I called for the appointment, I asked what the doctor was like. The woman I spoke

to said he was about sixty years old, very easy to talk to, and a wonderful surgeon. She had been with him for thirty years and he had
performed breast-cancer surgery on her too! His practice was about
80 percent breast surgery. I envisioned a kindly little old man. I felt
reassured.

Again, I went alone. My biggest surprise was that this kindly "little old man" was tall, attractive, and personable. I could not help
thinking that I really must be getting old if sixty looked this good!
What's more, he was very straightforward and willing to give me any
level of information I wanted. I told him something that day that
pretty much summed up the way I was feeling about the whole situation. Logically, I knew all the statistics and survival rates, but the reality of breast cancer for me was my mother's experience. Even though
my brain told me to be positive, my emotions were reliving her death.

He told me what I already knew: that it had to come out. He
explained that I was a good candidate for lumpectomy with radiation because of the size and location of the lump—it appeared to be
a little over one centimeter and was in the upper quadrant, close to
the surface. He offered me the option of a simple mastectomy without radiation or a lumpectomy with radiation. For me, it was a no-
brainer. Given an option of keeping the breast, I took it. According
to the doctor, the survival rates were just as good and the surgery
much easier, even though I would have to endure seven weeks of
radiation. The surgery was scheduled for the following week, on
May 5.

Now I had to break the news to Alison and figure out how to
handle work and my closet business. That evening I called my
daughter. She was frightened, but held together and said she would
come down from Charleston the night before the surgery and stay as
long as I needed her. My sister was planning to fly in from Memphis
for the surgery. I also called my niece (actually my ex-husband's
niece), whom I had practically raised and had remained very close to.

She, too, was quite frightened, but said she would be at the hospital. And she generously offered to pick up my sister at the airport and bring her to the hospital the morning of the surgery.

I decided to take the "chicken" way out at work. I could not really talk about what was happening without breaking down and crying, and could not deal with others' reactions or questions just yet. I decided to tell only my manager and three people with whom I worked closely, and not let anyone else know. For me it was easier to go to work and put the cancer aside for those eight hours. If everyone knew, I would have to deal with questions all day, and at that point I had more questions than answers. I sent an e-mail late that afternoon to the four people I had chosen to tell, letting them know what was going on and asking that they not tell anyone else for now. They were all very supportive. My boss set things up for me to work from home (at my request) and told me to do whatever I needed. I spent the next few days at work getting things arranged so that my responsibilities would be covered while I was out for surgery, and so that I could work from home as soon as possible.

That weekend was spent cleaning house and taking care of pending issues in my business. On Monday, Rick came down with an intestinal virus and was totally absorbed in his own misery. When I got home from work on Tuesday, he was lying on the bed acting perfectly pitiful. Alison was due in around eight o'clock that evening, and I was in no mood to baby Rick at that point. He asked if I wanted him to stay with his parents so that I would not catch whatever he had. I quickly said yes.

I put on jeans and went to the barn. I saddled Magnum for what I was afraid would be the last time, but hoped, just the last time for a while, and we headed out. I kept thinking that Magnum had always been there for me when I needed him most, which at that point, was a lot more than I could say for Rick. I was furious at him for bailing out on me, but could not say anything because he was legitimately sick. I also admit that I believed then, as I do now, that he did not have a contagious virus, but rather, had made himself physically ill from the anxiety of not knowing how to deal with my cancer. I did not feel the least bit sorry for him either. When I got back from riding, he was gone and my daughter had just driven up. We spent a tense evening planning for the next few days. Alison was obviously nervous but remained upbeat, which helped keep me from dwelling on my fears.

I was to report to the Atlanta hospital at 9:00 a.m. Living as far out of the city as I do, and allowing for morning rush-hour traffic, we left home at 7:00 a.m. and still arrived a little late. The two hours of heavy traffic did nothing to calm my nerves. I went through several hours of pre-op, and when I was finished, I returned to the waiting room where my sister and niece were waiting. After a while, I was taken to radiology for the ultrasound-guided insertion of a wire into the lump. It was uncomfortable but not painful. However, anxiety had definitely set in. After the wire was in place, another mammogram was done to confirm correct placement. That mammogram was probably the most painful part of the entire surgery. After I had changed into the fashionable surgical garments, my sister, daughter, and niece came back to see me before I was taken to the operating room. I told each of them I loved them and we all tried unsuccessfully not to cry. Once in the O.R., I remember looking up at the lights and telling God that I was turning the rest over to him. That was the last thing I remember until I woke up in recovery.

When they wheeled me to my room, Marian and Alison were there. Alison had brought me a fuzzy teddy bear named "Harry." I smiled and hugged Harry and then fell asleep for most of that afternoon and evening. Rick came by for a while (I am not sure how long, thanks to the drugs), and then he headed home to take care of the horses. Phil was out of town on business and called me at the hospital that evening. My sister left to spend the night at my niece's house, and Alison and I settled in for the night. Around ten o'clock, the nurse came in to empty the drain from the incision. She was a little rough, and the pain went all the way into my shoulder and back as she drained it. After she left I started feeling lightheaded. Alison asked if I was all right. I said no and pushed the call button at the same time that she headed to the nurses' station to get help. Then, I fainted. When I opened my eyes, I had needles going into my arm and about ten people were milling around my bed in a near panic. I could not figure out why everybody was so excited over a simple fainting spell. Evidently, when they had gotten to me, I had no pulse or blood pressure. A male nurse in the hallway saw Alison's face and immediately ran into my room, not even asking Alison if anything was wrong. It was his face I saw when I came to. Once I was awake and my vital signs got back to normal, I settled in for the night, albeit under closer supervision than before. By morning, I was doing better and the doctors decided that I had experienced a "vagal nerve" reaction, which temporarily arrests respiration. I still just felt like I had fainted, but it certainly got everyone's attention. My surgeon came in after lunch and told me that I could go home or stay another night. Home was definitely preferable! In fact, I felt pretty good and actually fed the horses by myself that night. I was encouraged that I was able to get back to "life on the farm" and take care of myself so quickly.

My sister left the next day and Rick came back to the house. I spent the rest of the week and weekend resting. I was bored, but I decided not to go back to the office until after the drain was removed. My breast was sore and looked scary with all the staples in it, but at least it was still *there*. Alison stayed a few days and went home on Sunday. I was very grateful for her visit. Early the next week, I went back to see the surgeon and get the pathology results. He had "good" news and "other" news that took some digesting. The nodes were negative. That was the "biggie" in my mind. The tumor was estrogen positive (but only 10 percent), progesterone positive (90 percent), the S phase was fairly high, and one of the two DNA types was an aggressive type. Estrogen positive and progesterone positive indicates that the tumors are sensitive to hormones and are usually slower growing. The S phase is a measurement of the percentage of cells that are dividing at a given time. A higher S phase indicates a more aggressive cancer. By now, I was approaching information overload. My surgeon recommended an oncologist, and I made yet another doctor's appointment.

The oncologist had ordered a "HER2/neu" test when he had received my records. After a lot of questions and conversation, I left with the understanding that if the test came back positive, I would need radiation and chemotherapy; if it was negative, I would only need radiation. The HER2/neu test is a predictor of aggressive cancers. I really sweated the results of that one. I was deathly afraid of chemotherapy since my mother had actually died from the effects of the chemo (at least in my mind). Alison asked if I wanted her to come to Atlanta to be with me when I got the final results. My first instinct was to refuse. I reasoned that asking her to travel all that way just to attend one doctor's visit was unnecessary. However, for once in my life, I answered honestly by telling her that it would mean a lot to have her with me. She drove back to Atlanta the following week and we went to my oncologist for the results. Alison was my "second set of ears." I was so emotional, I tended to have selective hearing. Having my daughter there helped me to keep all the information, not just what I chose to hear. As soon as we sat down, the doctor said he had good news. The HER2/neu was negative. I was so relieved I almost didn't hear what he said next. He said that since the test was negative, I would be able to take CMF (Cytoxan/methotrexate/5-fluorouracil) chemotherapy instead of AC (Adriamycin/Cytoxan). My response was that he could not be right. My nodes were negative, this new test was negative; I should not have to have chemotherapy. He explained that, unfortunately, when all of the factors balanced, he still recommended chemo, primarily because of my age, family history, the tumor size, and the S phase. Almost everything in my case was *borderline*. He said that in premenopausal women, chemo was indicated, but in postmenopausal women, tamoxifen appeared to be as effective. Since I was "perimenopausal," that put me right on the fence. He would not insist on the chemo, it would be up to me. He referred me to a female radiation oncologist, and I set up yet another doctor's appointment.

Now I really felt like I was carrying the weight of the world. I had to make what could be a life-or-death decision and did not have any clear guidelines. I spent a long time discussing my predicament with the radiation oncologist, who was absolutely wonderful. She had the same kind of family history I did and knew firsthand the fears. Her mother had taken CMF, and she was able to give me a great deal of insight into the reality of those particular drugs. She ultimately recommended I take it, but agreed that it was a gray area and the decision would have to be mine. I finally decided that since the "perimenopausal/postmenopausal" placement seemed to be a marker of sorts, I would talk to my gynecologist and try to find out where I actually fit at that point in time. He took a blood test that would give us a better idea and, for once, something came back definitive. I was absolutely premenopausal. Okay, not a good answer for avoiding chemo, but at least a concrete guideline.

Now for the really tough decisions. I was someone who had always felt that I could handle anything life threw at me. I never would have believed that, one day, I would find myself in a situation where I would need group or individual therapy. But here I was, needing information and support, and not wanting to burden my family. I had received some information from the hospital, after my surgery, about The Wellness Community, the organization that provided support for cancer patients. I called their telephone support contact and spent a good bit of time on the phone with her over the next couple of days. It was amazingly helpful to talk to someone who had actually been where I was and had survived. I also got information about The Wellness Community's breast-cancer support group. I had never been to a support group of any kind in my life. My standard "M.O." was to tough things out by myself. But this was bigger than anything I had ever had to deal with. I decided to give The Wellness Community a try and see if anyone there had experiences similar to mine. I think I was really looking for someone to tell me it was okay to refuse the chemo.

It felt very awkward to sit in a room full of strangers and discuss such intensely personal issues, but the warmth and understanding was overwhelming. I came away that first day still fighting the chemo decision, but feeling not quite so alone. I learned that it was easier (not easy, but easier) to talk to people who were *not* close to me because the caretaker in me did not want to hurt my family. And these discussions hurt. At the end of each group meeting, the facilitator had everyone stand in a circle, hold hands, close their eyes, and breathe deeply for a couple of minutes. As I was standing there, holding hands with total strangers, I actually felt an electric current go through my body from each hand I was holding. It startled me so much that I flinched. I am still convinced that the emotional healing in that group is almost palpable. As a long-standing member of The Wellness Community group, I now try to stand next to new members in the circle and transfer "positive" energy to them, as the group did for me in the beginning.

The women in my support group had helped me realize that there really is "life after chemo." But everything I knew firsthand about chemotherapy was from the few people I knew personally who had taken it. None had survived. Within the support group, I met women who led happy, productive lives during and after chemo. Later, in the course of treatment, after more of my friends learned of my diagnosis, I found that I actually knew a number of people who had been through treatment. I just was not aware of it. I was encouraged and put the decision-making behind me, ready to tackle the task at hand.

I had only one major reservation left to resolve. For years, I have had mild to moderate pain in my lower back (near the sacroiliac joint), which I have attributed to arthritis or just plain getting old. The pain was in the exact spot where my mother's cancer had recurred. Before beginning chemotherapy, particularly since I would be taking the less severe drugs, I talked to my oncologist about the back pain. He suggested that I have a bone scan to rule out the possibility that there was any malignancy there. Once I knew that there was cancer in my body, it was hard *not* to imagine that every little pain could be more cancer. The bone scan indicated that it was indeed arthritis, and we scheduled the first chemotherapy treatment for late June.

I had a two-closet installation the weekend prior to the first treatment, which would finish up my pending jobs. Unfortunately, due to builder delays, Rick and I were only able to complete one of the two closets prior to chemo. The second one would have to be installed on Sunday, two days after my first round of chemo. Not knowing how I would react to the drugs, I was concerned about my ability to do the physical work required to complete the task. I decided to ask my niece's husband if he would come and help us install it on Sunday. He agreed and the three of us were able to finish it on schedule, thank goodness. One less bit of stress and responsibility to deal with! This was the first of my many lessons in allowing others to help out. I finally learned to accept offered help graciously, and to understand that it also helped my friends because they were able to do something to show their concern for me.

The doctors delayed the beginning of radiation until after my first cycle of chemo (radiation and chemo can be given concurrently when taking CMF). I asked the radiation oncologist to give me tattoos so I would not have to deal with the markers and tape during the waiting period and radiation. After all, it was summer and the farm still had to be taken care of. Tape, ink, and sweat on my chest for the entire summer did not strike me as attractive. The tattoos were five, tiny, blue dots that were barely noticeable.

I have a very close friend who is a critical care obstetric nurse at the hospital where I had the surgery. Pam and I are horse buddies from way back. I had told her about the cancer before the surgery, and she came to check on me at the hospital after surgery. When I decided to proceed with chemotherapy, she insisted on coming with me for the first treatment and staying with me that night. Rick had said nothing about taking time from work to go with me, and I was too stubborn to ask him to do so. I was grateful to have Pam offer to "baby-sit." I trust her explicitly as a friend and a nurse.

Just before the treatment began, Pam and I met with the doctor. He explained the drugs that would be used and the purpose of each. He also gave me prescriptions for nausea medication. I was very nervous and frightened, but having Pam there kept me a little distracted. The nurses at the clinic were well prepared for a patient's "first treatment anxiety" and went out of their way to explain things and check on me frequently. We sat in recliners in a corner of the large treatment room, and Pam kept me talking about other things (mostly horses). The drugs were administered by IV and took a little over two hours to complete. After the treatment, we went grocery and pharmacy shopping, trying to get home before the premedication wore off. When we got back home, I still felt good and actually had more energy than I needed. I went out to feed the horses and clean the barn. Then it occurred to me that the "buzz" of energy I felt was due to the steroid in the premeds. Pam and I had a fun "girls' evening," cooking dinner, watching movies, and doing manicures. She had a tennis match the next day, so I talked her into leaving in time to make it. I was obviously not going to have a problem with the nausea and felt perfectly comfortable staying home by myself. I tried to just take it easy over the weekend, and worked from home on Monday as planned. Rick had come back to the house on Saturday, and we fell back into our regular routine.

When I went back for blood counts the next week, they were down but not dangerously low. The oncologist cleared me to start radiation right before the next chemo treatment was scheduled. I asked him about dropping the steroid premed because I did not appear to need it to prevent nausea. Besides, I really disliked the "buzz" it caused, and I have an aversion to taking steroids anyway. The doctor seemed surprised that I would want to drop it, but was willing to do so. I also asked if he would change the nausea premed to another drug because I had gotten intense headaches the week after treatment—a common side effect of that particular drug. I appreciated his willingness to let me take part in the decisions surrounding the treatment. I think my expectation was a somewhat dictatorial approach to treatment on the part of the doctor, but I got just the opposite.

As planned, I worked from home on Monday and returned to the office on Tuesday as if nothing had happened. I worked a slightly shorter day and continued to work from home one day a week. After a couple of weeks, I realized that I was getting very tired by the middle of the week. I made the decision (with my manager's full support) to sleep as late as possible and come in to work at whatever time I got there. My body was demanding more rest than normal.

As I settled into a routine of chemo and work, I did not make many concessions in my lifestyle other than allowing myself more rest. I was determined not to let the treatments dictate what I could and could not do. The one concession I did make was to give up my evening glass of wine. My oncologist had said that an occasional glass of wine would not hurt, but not to drink excessively. Since I tend to be drug-sensitive, I decided that it would probably be in my best interest to cut out alcohol entirely. However, I really missed drinking a glass of wine while I was cooking dinner. Finally, I came up with a solution that allowed me to have the drink without risking a reaction. I mixed what I dubbed a "Chemo Cocktail" and sipped on it while cooking. It was served in a wine glass or frosted mug and contained cranberry juice, orange juice, and Sprite. It satisfied my need for a "drink," and I did not even miss the alcohol.

I started attending weekly support group meetings at The Wellness Community. This was my time to talk about what was going on in my body and my head. I still could not seem to talk to anyone else about it with any degree of depth or detail. My instinct was to put up a good front, to protect those around me whom I loved. Unfortunately, that meant I kept it all inside. The Wellness Community group gave me the outlet and the support I needed from people who were in the same boat as I was. It was also a wonderful place to learn things you would not learn in a doctor's office. Even though my doctors were great about answering my questions, it was the group that helped me know *what* to ask.

My radiation treatments started the week before my second round of chemotherapy. The technicians at the clinic were friendly and upbeat, and the treatment itself was painless. At their suggestion, I was using natural aloe (from the plant) twice each day on the breast to help prevent burning. The biggest negative was the commute to the clinic every day. I had scheduled my daily appointments during lunch time to avoid morning or evening rush-hour traffic. Although my working days were pretty normal, the midday interruption was a constant reminder that I had cancer. One of the things that I had learned from the very first woman I spoke with at The Wellness Community was about visualizations. She described the visualization that she used during radiation. The treatment only lasts about a minute, but it can be a very long minute. I worked on a visualization tailored to my life and came up with one centered on my new dog, Sadie. She's an Australian shepherd and will herd anything that moves. At the time of my surgery, she was only five months old and a real handful. Fortunately, her energy level kept me moving, too.

My visualization was as follows:

Sadie and I were standing side by side at the edge of a field (my breast). As soon as the radiation began, I sent her out and she circled the entire mass, barking and nipping at cancer cells to herd them under the radiation beam. When the machine clicked off, I called her back to my side.

Being the very practical, down-to-earth person that I am, I never would have thought I could benefit from a visualization technique. But I certainly did! It made me feel less like a victim and more like a survivor, and gave me a small sense of control over a situation that often seemed totally out of my control.

Somewhere in the middle of the seven weeks of radiation, I had a unique, transforming experience. I frequently had trouble concentrating on the visualization while the machine was running, but I pushed myself to try. One day while I was concentrating on Sadie going after the "bad" cells, I suddenly saw a large translucent hand reach down and with one finger push a stray cell up under the radiation beam. It was very real, and I believe that it was God's way of telling me (rather graphically) that He was there helping, too. I have continued to use the vision of His hand whenever I am praying for someone who is going through a difficult time. I concentrate on His hand cradling the person during surgery or whatever the particular difficulty is.

I expected to breeze right through the second chemo treatment just as I had the first. I drove myself to the clinic, and everything went smoothly. I did not take steroids this time, and felt better that afternoon than I had the first time around. I actually got some sleep that night. Rick was working the next day, so he left early in the morning. When I woke up around 9:00 a.m., I thought I had been hit by a train. I was not nauseous, but just felt so lousy that I could hardly walk. My face and chest were bright red. Sadie was full of energy and ready to play. I managed to take her outside briefly, but realized that I could not possibly cope with her all day. Nor could I make it out to the barn to put her in her day kennel. I called one of my neighbors for help, and she came and took Sadie out to the barn for me. I spent the rest of the day on the couch. Pam came by that afternoon to check on me and told me that the reaction was natural and was normally masked by the steroids, which apparently serve a purpose beyond preventing nausea. By the next day, I felt well enough to go to a horse show with Pam to see her stallion perform. Each successive day, I felt a little bit better. When I went back to the clinic for my blood counts, they were still holding at a safe level.

The nurse practitioner at the radiation clinic gave me some good advice when I mentioned my aversion to taking steroids and what had happened after the last chemo treatment. She suggested I cut the dose in half to see if it might strike a happy medium between the two reactions. She also convinced me that a very small dose would simply be passed through the body, unlike some of the steroid injections that are used in joints. I took her advice and it worked beautifully. I did not get the jitters the first day and only a slight rash by the end of the second day.

Over the course of the six chemo treatments, my blood counts dropped below the danger threshold only twice. The first time, the oncologist delayed the treatment for a week and my counts rebounded on their own. The second time, he prescribed Neupogen injections to keep the counts up because it was later in the treatment cycle and he was not sure they would rebound on their own quickly enough. The injections were not as bad as I had anticipated.

Pam came over the first couple of days and taught me how to do them. She also brought some smaller needles, which made the process much easier. For the most part, I let Rick inject me, but at least I knew I could do it by myself if I needed to. I had given my horses shots all the time, but it is a little different when it's your own body.

One of the biggest fears and hurdles to get past when facing chemotherapy is hair loss. Even though I had been told that most people only lose part of their hair when taking CMF, I was still very apprehensive about it. In a discussion at The Wellness Community group meeting, one of the women related a method to prevent, or at least minimize, hair loss that she had tried when she was taking chemo. She had some success with it, so I decided it was worth a try. It sounds a bit comical, and in fact *is* quite comical, but I was desperate. The theory is that if you pack your head with ice packs during the administration of the IV drugs, the hair follicles are not as affected and, therefore, there is less hair loss. For my second or third treatment I decided to go for it. I took a cooler of crushed ice in plastic bags to the clinic with me. I also took along a beige towel to wrap around my head once I got everything positioned. And, yes, I did look ridiculous. I guess the nurses in the chemo room have seen everything because no one actually laughed or even seemed curious. A word of caution: it is not easy to get ice packs to stay on your head for any length of time, and they get *very* cold. When I settled into a recliner for the treatment that day, I looked at the woman in the chair next to me who was curled up asleep with an IV drip in her arm. I couldn't see her face very well but she looked like one of the women I had met at my support group. After I got settled, got my head wrapped, and had the drugs started, she stirred a bit and I called her name. She slowly looked at me with an odd expression on her face, and after a minute she recognized me and we talked for a while. She was having a very hard time recovering from her first AC treatment and had come in for IV fluids. She couldn't drive and didn't know how she was going to get home, so I offered to drive her home after we both finished up. She later told me that when she awoke and saw me that day, she could only see my face and a pale yellow glow around it. She thought I was an angel. I have been called a lot of things in my life, but "angel" was a new one!

When I still had a few radiation treatments and several chemo treatments to go, my ninety-five-year-old aunt (and breast-cancer survivor) died. I postponed the last few radiation treatments and a chemo treatment to go to her funeral. My sister and I were her closest relatives, so we were handling all the arrangements. My daughter went with me on the seven-hour drive to Tennessee. We got there just in time for me to take a short nap before going to the funeral home. The long trip was tiring (I did all the driving) and unbearably hot, but I made it without any of my own physical problems getting in the way, and was very glad I had gone.

Shortly after I had finished radiation treatments, and about midway through the chemo, my manager planned a team building outing to go white-water rafting. I loved to raft and decided to give it a shot. My doctor approved as long as my blood counts were high enough, so I signed up. I even volunteered to drive a carload of people up to the Ocoee River (it was more than a two-hour drive). We left early and planned to run the river twice—a two-hour run each time. It was August and the weather was good that day, warm enough to keep us from freezing in the river. When we grouped off for the rafts, I found myself quickly surrounded by my manager and the other three people on the trip who knew about my illness. I had been a little apprehensive about being in a raft without anyone knowing, just in case something happened. They solved that problem without ever saying a word. No one babied me, but it was comforting to know that they were there if I needed them. We had a great time, but as we stepped into the river for the second run, I remember thinking, *What am I doing? I'll never make it through a second time!* But I did. Although I was extremely tired at the end of the day and thought we would never get home, I had a renewed sense of confidence, of being able to "take charge," of doing the physical things I loved. At that point in my treatment, I needed the reassurance that I could still live life the way I always had—full speed ahead.

According to the original schedule, my last chemo treatment was to be Thanksgiving weekend. Due to the two delays over the course of treatment, it was scheduled instead for the first week in December. My daughter had been home for Thanksgiving Day. The following day she and her husband left to visit other family. Rick also left that morning to go hunting for the weekend. I had planned to load the horses and meet some friends to camp and ride for two days. Because of rain, I delayed the decision to go until late that morning, but finally decided to pack up and go. As I walked toward the bedroom, I tripped over a rug and fell into the couch, trying to catch myself with my right hand. When I hit the floor, everything hurt, but especially my right wrist. I lay there alone and cried, mostly out of frustration. I finally got up and hobbled to the bathroom to wrap my wrist. Camping was pretty much out of the question at that point since I could not even lift my saddle to put it in the truck, much less get it on a horse's back. I was so angry with myself and miserable that I cried most of the afternoon. When I saw my oncologist for my last chemo treatment the following week, he suggested an X-ray. My wrist turned out to be fractured. I spent the next four weeks in a cast and several weeks afterward in a brace. I was beginning to wonder if the physical setbacks would ever end.

The weekend before my last treatment, I had another closet installation scheduled. This was a big job and, unfortunately, I had to do it with an injured wrist. But, at least by now I knew my body's cycles with the chemotherapy and was able to schedule my work accordingly. The job went well and we finished on time despite my slight handicap. I had somehow managed to install one closet two days after my first treatment, several during treatment, and another one two days before my last treatment.

My last chemo treatment was coming up and I was anxiously awaiting the day. As it drew nearer, Rick mentioned that he was planning to leave on Thursday to go deer hunting for a few days. My last treatment was on Friday, and I guess I had expected him to understand how important that milestone was to me. When I reminded him, he was encouraging and happy for me, but did not offer to cancel his hunting trip to go with me and share the celebration. I did manage to convey to him my disappointment that he had forgotten about my final treatment and what it meant to me. But a-hunting he went anyway. The day before that final treatment, Phil called to congratulate me on nearing the "finish line." He offered to go with me to the clinic, and take me out to lunch to celebrate afterward. I gratefully accepted.

Finally, I was through with chemo! There was, however, one small glitch. I knew I was having some balance problems and that it probably had contributed to my fall at Thanksgiving. When I told my oncologist, he suggested that I have a CAT scan, just to be sure there was nothing unusual going on in the brain that could be causing it. Another, brand-new fear to deal with.

The nurse scheduled the CAT scan for the following week. When she called with the results, she said they looked good, but there was one small area that was slightly suspicious. They wanted to follow it up with an MRI. I no longer took these tests in stride and now was scared to death. I had told Rick about the CAT scan results, but, again, he had trouble remembering the scheduled MRI. Phil offered to go with me, and I accepted because I knew that, this time, I would have the results a couple of hours after the test and I did not want to be alone. Fortunately, the results were favorable. Rick finally remembered to ask about it a few days later.

So, the treatments were over and my life could get back to its regular pace. I guess I expected that I would instantly feel normal again. I was lucky that I had only lost about half my hair, and what was lost would eventually grow back. I did not look much different than when this whole nightmare had begun. Of course, I certainly *felt different inside*. Christmas came and went and I still did not have my old energy back. It actually took about three or four months before I even began to approach the energy level needed to tackle life the way I had always before. It has been a slow trip, but I'm getting there.

The final part of my treatment plan was a five-year course of tamoxifen. My aversion to drugs included this one. During my one-month post-treatment visit, my oncologist brought it up and said that he would let it be my choice to take the drug or not. My tumor was only 10 percent estrogen positive (90 percent progesterone positive), and tamoxifen is only effective on estrogen positive cancers. Translated, this meant that the effectiveness of the drug was directly related to the positive percent of the tumor. I grabbed the chance to avoid taking it. But later, I reconsidered this decision, and I discussed it with my oncologist a second time. He explained that he did not insist on my taking it because I had already had radiation and chemotherapy, and he did not feel that the additional treatment was really necessary. Tamoxifen is a chemo drug and is used to treat existing cancers, as well as prevent new breast cancers. He said that if I wanted to take it as a preventive, I was certainly a candidate. I came to the conclusion that even though this tumor was only 10 percent estrogen positive, given my family history, the likelihood of another cancer was pretty high. And the next tumor might be different. So, as much as I hated the idea, I went ahead with the tamoxifen. At least if I did have a recurrence, I would know that I had done everything I could to prevent it. Many members of the support group take tamoxifen, so I was able to get a pretty good picture of the side effects. Ironically, they are very much the same as menopause. It just exacerbates the weight gain, hot flashes, and mood swings. My oncologist has been very helpful in trying to find ways to minimize the side effects. I am taking a very low dose of Zoloft, an antidepressant, and using a Catapres patch to combat the hot flashes. I have completely cut caffeine out of my diet. The Zoloft also helps ease the mood swings, but probably contributes to the weight gain.

Rick no longer lives with me, but we maintain a friendly relationship. I was finally able to tell him how I felt about the way he dealt with (or didn't deal with) my cancer. I needed so much more from him than he could give, but I also realize now that it was unfair to expect things of him without letting him know what they were. I try to keep that in perspective and learn from it, enjoying the good parts of the relationship and not dwelling on the bad.

Since my diagnosis, my illness has taught me a lot about myself and those around me. I have learned that the love and support of my family and friends and my faith in God are the keys to surviving and making a better life after cancer. My sister and my daughter have been my anchor—sadly, my cancer has drastically increased their odds of facing the same fate some day.

I have learned a lot about what is really important in life and hope that I can keep that in focus as I continue the journey.

Above all, I have learned that I am not bulletproof . . . but with the love and support of my family, the help of The Wellness Community, and my support-group buddies, I have bulletproof armor if I need it.

Beth was thrilled when her daughter and son-in-law moved back to the Atlanta area from Chicago. And, she is now the proud grandmother of a baby boy. Beth also has a new addition to her animal family—a colt. Her cancer remains in remission.

Selden McCurrie

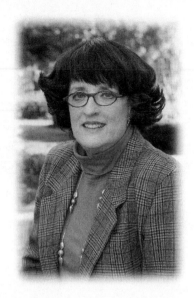

is an information development consultant in Atlanta, Georgia. She writes, edits, and produces documentation, Web content, and online help for software products. She earned a bachelor's degree in journalism and has taken graduate courses in Business Administration. In honor of her parents, she founded two scholarships at the universities they had attended, and cofounded a third one in honor of her undergraduate journalism professor. She serves on the board of directors for the latter scholarship and is proud that it has, to date, helped six young people get their degrees in communication. Selden loves to read, garden, and go antiquing.

DIAGNOSIS PROFILE

Age at diagnosis:	50 years old
Family history:	Mother, breast cancer at age 78
	Second cousins, breast cancer in their 80s
Symptoms:	None—abnormal mammogram
Surgery:	Bilateral mastectomy
Biopsy results	
Left breast:	DCIS
	Solid & cribriform patterns with necrosis
	Stage: 0
	Tumor size: 1.8 cm
	Grade: 3
Right breast:	Infiltrating ductal carcinoma
	Stage: 1c
	Tumor size: 1.2 cm
	Grade: 2
	Nodes: Sentinel node on right negative

Courage is the price that life extracts for granting peace.
—Amelia Earhart

Eyes on the Prize

SELDEN McCURRIE

On July 29th I was initiated into a vast unwilling sisterhood—I was diagnosed with breast cancer. I paced back and forth, cordless phone clutched in hand so tightly my knuckles were white as I waited for my doctor to come on the line.

My husband, Sam, was working from home, hunched over his laptop that Tuesday afternoon as the blinding July sunlight streamed through the bay window in the den. Our golden retriever, Harry, a precious fur child, though a poor substitute for our childlessness, snoozed in oblivion on the sofa. I watched dog hair waft by the ceiling fan.

"I'm sorry, Selden." My doctor's husky voice was inordinately gentle. "You have cancer in both breasts. The left breast shows extensive ductal carcinoma in situ, almost three centimeters. The right is infiltrating ductal carcinoma, around a centimeter. They're both highly treatable, though I'd like it better if the right wasn't infiltrating. I've taken the liberty of making an appointment with a surgeon for you. I'll fax you the biopsy results."

I mumbled thanks and hung up. Tears in my eyes, I turned to face Sam. He hugged me as I buried my face in his chest. We swayed together into a pool of sunlight. The light warmed the cold pit of dread that was forming in my stomach. Harry bounced off the sofa to sit at our feet.

"Remember, they've caught this early," Sam said, resting his chin on the top of my head, his beard tickling my forehead, his hands massaging my back. "We'll get through this together. Go ahead and let yourself cry, it will do you good." In the background I could hear the fax machine whine in my upstairs office.

"I'll cry about this tomorrow. I want to see the biopsy reports. We've got to hit the ground running." I forced myself to compartmentalize my feelings, a blessing or a curse that had served me well in my fifty years. To take a deep breath and let the intellect take over, then move into data collection mode. Slap a notepad in my hand and get a Pavlovian response—I become a reporter again. Do the work, get the story, then give in to my emotions.

As I padded upstairs, I dodged our sixteen-year-old cat, Arthur, on the top step as I tried to count the times I had played this scene in my head. Were these biopsies numbers six and seven or five and six? There had been so many over the years, not counting the needle aspirations. So many mammograms and ultrasounds. I remembered my first baseline mammogram when I was in my twenties. I had plopped my breast on an X-ray table and the technician packed sandbags around it.

I remembered the recent mammograms and the "thrill" of having my D-cup breasts compressed. This year, they had done magnification films, a first for me. My breast was compressed with a hollow circular paddle the size of a tennis ball, and I immediately let out a string of obscenities—it hurt. Barb, the technician (she was known affectionately as "Barb the Butcher"), was a master at ferreting out the tiniest blip with her magnification films. She had a gift for early detection.

I remembered the ultrasounds and watching the monitor as the technician moved the sensor over my breasts. The images always reminded me of bubbles, like the ones I had blown as a kid. A little more pressure and a bubble would part, if it was benign. If it didn't, it was solid and had to be biopsied. Two different technicians and three tries had found the tumor in the right breast. Only the slightest difference between this year's mammograms and last year's had led them to the area. And this year, one bubble didn't part—the tumor in my right breast.

My breasts were dense and fibrocystic. I had had complex cysts aspirated. I had ducts biopsied because of ductal proliferation, which meant the cells were multiplying. Core biopsies were performed with a device that looked like a gun and could have only been designed by a man. And now a week earlier, a stereotactic biopsy. Lying on a table with my breast in a compression vise, while my doctor used a digitized mammogram and computer to guide her to the spot to biopsy.

Through all these procedures, I had developed a pattern of coping. Compulsively, I would begin researching *breast cancer* as soon as I got home from the doctor's office. Know your enemy was my motto. If you knew your enemy well enough, you could find the weapons to defeat it and manage your fear. I had all but memorized the breast cancer bible: *Dr. Susan Love's Breast Book*. I thanked God for the modern technology that made Medline, the National Institute of Health's database of medical publications, accessible from home. I was grateful for my four years of medical software experience, which gave me some ability to decipher the information that my queries turned up.

The medical party line statistics said I was a sitting duck for breast cancer. Early menstruation at age ten, no pregnancies in twenty-one years of marriage, thirteen years on birth control pills to manage my endometriosis, and although my cycles were erratic, my single ovary was still pumping out estrogen at age fifty. Family history—my mother had breast cancer at seventy-eight, as did two of her cousins who were in their eighties when diagnosed. Three times I had waited with my father as she had undergone open biopsies, the kind where surgery is performed to remove the entire mass. Three times she had dodged a bullet. The last time it had hit when she had a core biopsy with the same physician who had diagnosed me.

I scanned the pathology reports. The cancer in the left breast was potentially fast growing, was killing cells, hence the areas of solid necrosis, but had not broken out of the ducts. The right breast had an infiltrating tumor with the greatest measurable dimension of 0.8 centimeters. No mention of vascularization, the tumor creating its own blood vessels, or of lymphatic involvement.

Not real good. Not real bad, but potentially nasty. As I walked back downstairs, I said a prayer for my husband. He had lost his mother to breast cancer when he was fifteen. Like me, she had had it in both breasts. Back in the late 1950s, they did not catch it until the large tumors had metastasized. Despite double radical mastectomies and cobalt radiation treatments, she had lasted five years only to die a gruesome death.

I wondered what he was thinking. He had held my hand through most of my previous biopsies. A scientist, who ironically was researching obscure properties of DNA at the molecular level where changes can cause malignancy, his real world knowledge of breast cancer was limited and theoretical.

"It doesn't look that bad," he said, scanning the reports. "This is why you've been going to doctors all these years, so they could catch it early. It's not an automatic death sentence."

He hugged me and I felt my breasts press against his chest, a pen in his pocket gouging my right breast. I stepped away.

"I want to rip these puppies off. I'm sick of going through this," I said, looking down at my breasts. It was the same thing I'd told my doctor while she was doing my stereotactic biopsy.

"Sel, I'll love you no matter what. Your breasts don't matter, as long as you're alive." I noticed that his eyes and nose were red. He'd been crying while I'd been upstairs. It was hard enough for me to suck it up and keep going, but I loathed the emotional hit on him.

I knew I was at the starting line of a race, a race not against time, but to *buy* time, because I knew the researchers were getting close to managing, if not curing, breast cancer. The prize was to get cancer-free and stay that way as long as possible. I was determined to keep my eyes on the prize.

* * * * *

I was once again entrenched in the medical world—a world unto itself. I had seen too much of what it had to offer over the span of my life. Endometriosis had bought me three laparoscopic surgeries and robbed me of my fertility. I had battled excruciatingly painful periods for years until the birth control pill had provided me with relatively normal college years. The last surgery at age thirty-nine to remove my right ovary had allowed me eleven pain-free years.

As an only child, I had comforted and helped my parents through their seven collective heart attacks, two heart bypasses, my father's colon cancer and surgery, his diabetes, my mother's carpal tunnel surgery, arthritis, and her breast cancer with subsequent mastectomy.

For well over ten years before their deaths, I jumped at phone calls in the middle of the night and early morning. I had kept a packed overnight bag in my car, complete with *Merck Manual*, a medical dictionary, and a prescription drug directory to help me decipher what the doctors would tell me in the Emergency Room or hospital.

I had another reason to be knowledgeable—my drug allergies. So far only hydrocodone could kill me, but others, like sulfa could make me violently ill. Unfortunately, there was no way to tell ahead of time if I was allergic to a drug. The reactions always showed up later. Even though all my doctors had my drug allergies well-documented on a sticker on the front of each of my files, I still checked. I only filled prescriptions at one pharmacy, had my allergies noted in the pharmacy database, and I kept a current *Physician's Desk Reference* and doubled-checked each new prescription.

I was medically militant—I wanted to know as much as possible, and I am sure some doctors disdained my endless questions. One doctor said to me, "You're a difficult patient. You ask hard questions and you challenge." My body, my life, my treatment. I had a right to know, and that was how I faced my fears.

But there was a price to pay for being medically militant: information overload. We had hit five doctors in two weeks. I had filled a notepad with questions, and we had a full complement of digitized audio CDs from our consultations.

Nights were the worst. Stress and the ever-increasing waves of hot flashes made sleep difficult. Things I had once found endearing now plucked at my tautly stretched control. Arthur, who slept curled around my head on the pillow, made this humid August night unbearable. I needed to make a decision soon. I prayed for wisdom. I prayed for strength.

I was trying to assemble an emotionally charged clinical jigsaw puzzle, but the pieces kept multiplying. Lumpectomies vs. mastectomies. Mastectomies were becoming a very real option. Mastectomies without reconstruction. "Reconstruction" was a term I had come to loathe for signifying that mastectomy was the ultimate de-construction. Implants were out because of my track record of allergies.

My history as a smoker meant a free flap TRAM was my only reconstruction option using my tissue—removing flaps of muscle from my abdomen and attaching them to my chest, then moving my belly fat to fashion breast mounds. It was a rigorous procedure with a long recovery period that could delay chemotherapy.

I wondered how easy detection would be with reconstruction. If the DCIS in my left breast ran to the chest wall, how could a surgeon be certain he had gotten it all? With reconstruction, I was told there would be no more mammograms, just yearly checks. How would a doctor know if the cancer came back?

Also, I knew it wasn't a question of if, but rather when, I would face a hysterectomy. Given my gynecologic track record, it was only a matter of time before something turned up. Although I hoped for a hysterectomy through the laparoscope, I knew that might not be possible. How easy would it be if I was reconstructed with a free flap TRAM? What would happen if they had to slit me from hip to hip to do a hysterectomy? Would that undo the tummy tuck part of the free flap? God forbid, but if I should need a heart bypass twenty years down the road, would that undo the reconstruction? Would I lose my breasts a second time?

Still, the major point was psychological. I couldn't handle reconstruction. At least not right away. I had seen a different type of reconstruction five years ago, and it haunted me to this day. My father, a diabetic, had a heart attack and subsequent quadruple coronary bypass surgery when he was eighty. His sternum—the bone in the center of his chest—had become infected and was removed. To protect his heart, he had had a flap done. In the days that followed, I stayed by his side and watched while nurses changed his bandages. I saw his flap pulsating with each beat of his heart. I had listened to his doctors debate the viability of the flap. "The flap looks pale today." "Uh—oh, its temp is down." The surgeon had been a master. The flap never failed—but my dad's heart did.

If I could shake the memories of my father's ordeal, reconstruction would always be an option. Nonetheless, I called our health insurance companies. If I wanted reconstruction at a later date, it would be covered but would require a letter of medical necessity from my doctor. I pondered that—letter of medical necessity. Losing your breasts to mastectomies wasn't enough on its own? What would make it a *necessity*? Nervous breakdown? Severe back problems?

For now, my choice was mastectomies without reconstruction vs. lumpectomies. I had wondered what mastectomies would be like, I thought as I tossed and turned, Sam's soft snores punctuating the dark silence of our bedroom.

I decided to go downstairs to the screened-in porch to sit. The quiet of the house enveloped me as I made my way in darkness. Making this decision was like groping in the dark.

"God's the only one who can tell me what to do here, and I don't think He's speaking directly to me now," I had moaned to Sam earlier that evening.

"Maybe not, but He's sending you women who will help you."

Statistics, studies, and medical opinions couldn't put a human face on mastectomies, so I wanted to go straight to the source. Early on, I had started going to a breast cancer support group at The Wellness Community. I felt an instant bond of sisterhood when I walked into the room.

These were the human faces behind the statistics. There were five women there that first day and I listened in awe as we went around the circle and told our stories. Theirs were the faces of choices: lumpectomy with radiation, lumpectomy with chemotherapy, mastectomy with reconstruction, and recurrence. Hope. These women were the embodiment of coping and hope. Yet there was no face for the choice of mastectomy *without* reconstruction.

I had put the word out that I was facing this decision and wanted to talk with women who had had double mastectomies—bilateral mastectomy in medical jargon. I discovered that this is the quietest group within this sisterhood to which I had been unwillingly initiated. There were women out there, granted not a lot, who were unreconstructed, but they were silent. I prayed for help. My prayers were answered.

Alice, a friend of a sister-in-law, called from her family's beach house one Sunday afternoon. Like me, she'd had cancer in both breasts. Unlike me, she had been a DD-cup before her mastectomies. She had forgone reconstruction. What's it like? I had asked.

"It's more comfortable than before and in fact, my back problems have gotten better," she said with a trace of a Boston accent. "I decided that I had to be consistent—either I was going to wear the prostheses all the time or not. So when I leave the house, I have them on. I hated the first prostheses and I loathed the mastectomy bras. I'm happier now that I've found this sports bra. It took some trial and error, so be sure you get measured by a certified fitter.

"I've lost part of my sexuality—my breasts, but my husband has been great. It will take you some time to get used to it."

Susan. I never knew how she found me—she left a message on my voice-mail. She told me she was a tall, athletic woman, and had also had a bilateral mastectomy without reconstruction.

"I was an A-cup before the surgery and now I can choose. For example, today, I wore B-cup prostheses, but tonight I'm going out and I'll wear C-cups. My insurance pays for a pair every year, so I've got several pairs. I like the ones that stick to your skin. They feel like a part of my body. I don't even think about it anymore," she said in a soft voice.

Jan, a geek like me—a computer project manager for a Fortune 500 company—also called one evening.

"I was small," Jan said. "I didn't even wear prostheses for the first two years. Nobody ever noticed. In fact, one day at work I mentioned my mastectomies to a programmer in the next cube who was a lean, tall, marathon runner. We stood side by side and you couldn't tell the difference. She was muscular and flat. I was short and flat.

"Then my husband started telling me my posture was changing. So I told him that for Christmas, I wanted a pair of boobs. I hit a department store that stocked prostheses and bought a pair. It did make a difference in my posture, and now I even wear them around the house."

Through the Internet, I had located mastectomy boutiques—shops that sell prostheses and mastectomy bras. One afternoon, I took myself to the local hospital's women's boutique.

"I may be having a bilateral mastectomy without immediate reconstruction and I'd like to look at the prostheses," I told the clerk behind the desk.

"Debbie's our fitter and she's with someone now. She'll be glad to help you if you care to wait," said the attractive, young clerk.

I nodded and sat down on a sofa to wait for the fitter. A few minutes later, a tall, beautiful, and completely bald woman sat down next to me. She was waiting for a wig fitting. She fished in her bag for a minute and brought out the latest bestseller, opened it, and began to read.

Trying not to be obvious, I glanced at her. This could be me in a few weeks—a chemotherapy patient. I absently twirled a strand of my hair and wondered if I would be so calm and serene while undergoing chemo. I had started prepping myself for chemo because I knew it was a possibility regardless of either surgical option.

Looking at the woman beside me, I remembered Lisa. Our paths had overlapped briefly before she moved out West to start what later became a multimillion-dollar consulting firm at the peak of the dotcom madness. We had stayed in touch through friends, and I had heard she was diagnosed with breast cancer years ago. When I received my biopsy results, I called her. She would be my touchstone if I got hammered with a cruel diagnosis.

"You'll get through it," Lisa said in her no-nonsense tone. "I did. Nine years out, despite having seven positive lymph nodes and being a Stage III, I'm doing fine. I look like a Picasso painting—the surgeon took out a big chunk of my breast. I gotta tell you, chemo was a little rough.

"I took a group of friends to each chemo session. We'd play cards and cut up while the stuff was dripping. I had it done on Thursday afternoons and was good until the next day, then I'd sack out for the weekend. I was able to get back to work by Monday, until they put me on some drug that started with a *V*. Screwed up my vision—couldn't watch TV or even read. I just ducked everything until I finished that.

"Make them tell you about lymphedema and go get fitted for a sleeve if they take out lymph nodes. I'd never even heard of lymphedema until I got it—I guess you heard about me breaking a collarbone when I got thrown from that mechanical bull. I got a personal trainer and a physical therapist, and now my arm is back to within 5 percent of normal. I may be late on my mortgage payments, but I won't skip my personal trainer. I train three days a week." When I hung up with Lisa, I knew I had a mentor in place.

The fitter, Debbie, a big-busted woman with a trim waist, was patient and showed me several types of prostheses. I held one in my hand and watched the silicon gel shift. We were standing in one of the private fitting rooms.

"It's very life-like and you can have it matched to your skin color," she said.

I juggled it from hand to hand and tried to imagine it next to my skin. Somehow, it seemed repugnant to me. It must have shown on my face because Debbie said, "I had a mastectomy eight years ago and chemotherapy. Have you thought about reconstruction?"

I explained that I wasn't sure.

"Want to see what a TRAM flap reconstruction looks like? I had mine done two years after my mastectomy." Her brown eyes were gentle.

Startled, I looked up and nodded.

"Lock the door," she said, unbuttoning her shirt.

I watched as she unhooked her bra. Her breasts were identical in shape and size. At a glance, there was no difference except the one on the left had no nipple and a faint web of scars on top.

She stood proudly before me and named the plastic surgeon who had done the work. He was the same one Sam and I had consulted.

"It's just the same as the other one but minus the nipple. I don't know if I'll have a nipple tatooed on it or not. Feel my tummy where they took the flap—it's like a tummy tuck," she said, dragging my hand to her belly. It was solid—no flab like me.

"It's beautiful," I said. "Thanks, I'll think about it."

I decided I was afraid of the prostheses—the silicon guys. In addition to my drug allergies, I had chemical sensitivities. I had already been tested for a latex allergy two biopsies back. The doctor did a core biopsy in the office and used a clear latex covering over the site. By the time I made it to the car, the skin under the bandage was burning.

One week, forty-plus scratch tests, and a couple of blood tests later, an allergist delivered the verdict.

"The only thing I can find that you're allergic to is your dog. I can't test you for adhesives or chemical sensitivities, but you're not allergic to latex."

"Harry isn't negotiable. He stays," I had said defiantly.

But now I worried that I *would* be allergic to prostheses. Flat forever. There must be alternatives to the silicon. I checked in with another mastectomy boutique that offered all types of lingerie and swimsuits.

I explained my plight to the sales clerk, a tall, slender, beautifully dressed woman named Annie.

"Let me show you other prostheses," she said, holding up two, soft big guys filled with something akin to pillow batting and covered with a T-shirt-like material. You could remove the batting, shaping them as you saw fit. Annie told me that many women wore these home from the hospital in a camisole.

I saw some "natural" prostheses, filled with something that rattled a little. I saw the stick-on prostheses with little ridges like suction cups. There were other options.

Somewhere around the third type, Annie told me that she had had a bilateral mastectomy without reconstruction.

"Almost five years out. I had it in my nodes and in my chest wall, but I'm okay now. I've worn all these different prostheses," she said.

I glanced at her. She had on a silk shirtwaist dress. I never would have thought she was wearing prostheses.

"I guess I'll take a pair of the big guys with a camisole," I said.

I tried on camisoles and cursed my broad shoulders.

"It's hard to gauge what size before your surgery," Annie said, bringing me an extra-large.

"How flat will I be? Should I get measured for a bra now? Would it make a difference?"

"Let me show you my incisions," Annie said as she stepped into the dressing room.

"See, I'm flat. Some women are so flat they're almost concave."

I looked. She had perfectly symmetrical scars and a smooth, flat chest, almost like a boy's.

Three surgeons were steering me toward bilateral mastectomy. Only the oncologist had said the survival odds at five years were the same for lumpectomies as mastectomies. A Mayo Clinic paper in Medline had turned up a slightly different outlook at ten years in favor of mastectomies. All four doctors had mentioned the hereditary potential of my cancer. In addition to my mother's breast cancer, my father had colon cancer at age seventy-eight. So had two of his brothers. I had had a colonoscopy in January so I knew I was clean. For now.

Back to assembling my clinical puzzle. My emotions nibbled at the edges of the pieces, making a good fit difficult. Where did my feelings go—in the middle or on the edges of the puzzle? And what were my feelings? Every time I thought about a bilateral mastectomy, I felt a sickening thud in the pit of my stomach. Yet, intellectually, I was leaning in that direction.

Snap. A genetic piece of the puzzle. My Medline queries had turned up papers implicating the hereditary aspects of breast cancer, which all my physicians had discussed with me.

Snap. A surgical piece of the puzzle. The surgeons who looked at my films, when pushed for an opinion on lumpectomies, had said it would be difficult to remove the entire duct. They could take the tumor out, but because of my dense, fibrous breasts could not be certain they would get the entire duct. I worried about what they could not see. The tumor was growing in a duct that had never been biopsied.

Snap. An anatomical piece of the puzzle. Breast cancer, especially DCIS, follows the duct. The oncologist said if I opted for lumpectomies, she would want to irradiate both breasts. Irradiation of my dense, heavy, elongated breasts, even with the best technology, carried a small chance of setting me up for potential heart disease. My mother had died of a heart attack—her seventh. I knew there were advances in radiation treatments, but I recalled a friend who had undergone radiation for his Hodgkin's disease, only to die twenty years later from leukemia. With mastectomies, at least I could duck radiation if the cancer wasn't in the lymph nodes.

Snap. A chemotherapy piece of the puzzle. We went to see the oncologist—a deceptively gentle woman whose businesslike demeanor hid a scientist's analytical mind. I walked away from her convinced she never forgot a single thing you ever told her. Despite multiple drug allergies and my complex medical history of chemical sensitivities, she was certain she could manage chemotherapy if I needed it. This hurdle was still an unknown—my final pathology report would determine whether or not I needed chemotherapy. I was operating under the assumption that I would. If not, then it would be a pleasant surprise.

Snap. A radiological piece of the puzzle. The radiologist who had diagnosed me said that only 40 percent of DCIS showed on mammograms. Who knew what else was cooking in my breast ducts?

Snap. A pathological piece of the puzzle. Most of what I read indicated that the woman most likely to get breast cancer was a woman who *had* breast cancer. If I chose lumpectomies, what were my odds of recurrence with cancer already in both breasts?

So much for medical and scientific opinions. Where did the human factors fit? How could I gauge what it would be like to lose my breasts? How would I know unless I had mastectomies? Would it be comfortable? Would I turn into the Hunchback of Notre Dame? If I had lumpectomies, would the cancer come back? Could I live with the stress of the three-month, six-month interval mammograms and ultrasounds? Could I face additional surgery? Did I want to gamble and take that chance? How would I handle all of this? How was I going to learn how to be a cancer patient?

I sat on the screened-in porch, in total darkness, with Harry curled on the floor beside my chair. I now owned my cancer, my enemy, and knew it well, but decided it would not *own* me. I closed my eyes and wished I could sleep. I prayed for guidance in making the decision. A hoot owl called in the distance. Was the owl a sign of dawning wisdom?

When I did sleep, I dreamed of breasts. Large breasts, small breasts. I surfed Web sites with photos of women who had mastectomies. Would that be me? During the day, when out and about, I found myself staring at women's breasts. I never noticed how many flat-chested women there were. I started wondering what it would be like to have no breasts. My big breasts had been with me since my teens. I remember at age twenty-two being voted "best bust in the newsroom" when I worked for a newspaper in those pre–sexual harassment days. Not to be outdone, the women reporters started voting, too. Best buns. The men retaliated with best legs. We voted best pects.

I remembered job interviews when I was a dress size 6 with a 36C bust and the male interviewers who would not take their eyes off my chest. I often retaliated by staring at their laps.

Once I had embraced computer geekdom, I seldom thought about how I looked. So long as I was neat and clean, what did it matter? It gave me a perverse sense of pride that I was accepted for my mind and my skills, not how I looked.

Sam would try and talk me through the anxiety attacks. This late night, he joined me on the porch.

"Sel, I'll love you no matter what. Parts or no parts. Your breasts and this breast cancer is just a tiny, tiny part of you and who you are. I just want you to live. I'll support whatever you choose," he said, looking up as he scratched Harry behind the ears.

"I'm hyperventilating over this," I whimpered. "I've got to make a decision, and I'm so scared of what can go wrong regardless of the surgery. It's not dying that I'm afraid of, it's what you go through before you die."

"You're stronger than you think you are. Look at your family. Remember your father at Pearl Harbor, your uncle at the Battle of the Bulge, and your uncle on the *USS Indianapolis*," Sam said.

I thought of my father. An Alabama farm boy who had enlisted in the Marines prior to World War II, he had been an anti-aircraft gunner on a ship. Just starting to dress for the last call for breakfast, when General Quarters sounded, my father fought the battle of Pearl Harbor in his skivvies. His ship had been damaged but stayed afloat. He had survived.

My uncle, who had been caught behind enemy lines during the

Battle of the Bulge, had been rescued by a French farm family. Day after day, he had stayed hidden in an attic until he could rejoin his unit. He had survived.

My other uncle floated in the Pacific after the *Indianapolis* had sunk, not knowing if rescue would come or not, while many of his shipmates died from shark attacks or their injuries. He had survived.

I remembered what my father once said to me on a rare occasion when he had talked about his experiences. "You have to trust God. There's only so much you can do. You have to put one foot in front of the other, keep going, and trust God." I knew that's what I had to do.

Sighing, I went back upstairs to try and catch a few hours' sleep. I was calmer as I climbed into bed, evicting Arthur who had taken my place. I plumped a pillow and settled in. Sam came to bed a few minutes later, and I felt a hand reach across the pillow for mine.

The painful realization dawned: bilateral mastectomy was my best option, but I wanted to see my radiologist one more time to ask about lumpectomies. I would have to live with my decision a long time. The only way I would have peace was to know all my questions had been answered.

"So what have you decided after your travels?" she said, walking into the examining room.

"I'm thinking about lumpectomies. Tell me how hard detection would be, given the way I scar?" I asked.

She clipped my mammograms on the light box, sighed, and turned to catch my eyes.

"If you want lumpectomies, we're here for you 24/7. We'd do mammograms and ultrasounds every six months for the rest of your life. But I want to tell you about a patient I had like you with cancer in both breasts. She chose lumpectomies and had chemo. She was fine until she developed ovarian cancer a few years later. Once again, she had surgery and did chemo. A few years after that, she developed breast cancer again, and even with careful monitoring, by the time we caught it, it was advanced. She died a few months later. Now I'm not saying that would be you. We can treat this breast cancer, but it's your potential for another breast cancer that I worry about. It's a chance you have to be willing to take."

"Thanks," I said with a sigh because she had crystallized what I had been afraid of. "I'm going to have a bilateral mastectomy."

The decision was made. I was ready to tell the family and friends who had been calling since the news of my diagnosis. I debated about going public with the mastectomies, but I decided if by being open, I could help one woman, even if it was through word of mouth, it would be worth it.

I told my brother-in-law one afternoon when he called. "You've got a great pair, but they ain't worth dying over," was his succinct response.

I told my family. Aunts and cousins called, offering their prayers and asking what they could do to help.

"Pray for the skill of my surgeon and pray for strength for me and Sam. That's the most important thing you can do for me," I told one aunt who called unexpectedly.

"We've been doing that all along. We love you and we won't stop praying for you," she said.

"I've got a broad shoulder to cry on if you need it, and I'll help you through chemotherapy," said another aunt who was undergoing chemo for her own cancer. "Just call me any time."

I told a friend, who was also a business colleague. When he and his wife adopted a child, I had filled in for him at his client meetings. When my parents became ill, he had filled in for me.

"You've been through enough. Oh God, why you?" he asked when I told him.

"Why not me? I'm no different from the thousands of women who are diagnosed every year," I snapped.

The anxiety escalated. Now I had to choose the surgeon. Five years earlier, I had chosen my father's cardio-thoracic surgeon for his heart bypass. He had been highly recommended and had done my mother's heart bypass eight years earlier. There had been terrible complications leading to my father's death, and I had always wondered if he would have survived had I chosen another surgeon. It was a question that still haunted me.

More than once I called my beloved cousin Amy in Alabama. Busy as she was caring for her disabled husband and a mother who had Alzheimer's, she would drop everything and pray with me when I called. I called this time and asked her to pray for me to choose the right surgeon. As we prayed together, I kept seeing the face of the last surgeon Sam and I had consulted.

The next day I telephoned this surgeon for an appointment.

First came a preoperative assessment. The more I saw of the surgeon, the calmer I felt. He spent almost an hour with us during this consultation, never once glancing at my page-long list of questions. He was a soft-spoken man, with years of experience, who exuded a strong sense of compassion and competence. He gave me the feeling that no matter what happened during surgery, he could handle it.

Armed with my ever-present notepad, I fired question after question at him. Never rushing me, he patiently answered, explaining every aspect of the surgery. When I told him I was scared, he grasped my hands, looked into my eyes and said, "I'll take good care of you."

I only had one question left on my list. "Any idea what my breasts weigh?" I asked.

The only clue that he hadn't been asked that question before was he blinked rapidly a couple of times before answering. "I don't know," he said.

"I'd like to know. Prostheses come in different weights. I figure I'll be most comfortable if I get a pair that approximate my breasts."

"I'll tell the pathologist to weigh them."

The mundane details of life went on. I did the weekly shopping, and as I carted a load of groceries to my car I felt a trickle of sweat run down my cleavage. I wondered what it would be like next summer with prostheses. Maybe I would tuck them in the fridge before I went out. They could keep me cool.

Physical activity held my anxiety at bay. I scrubbed and cleaned the house, preparing for the changes that would be required if I needed chemotherapy. Best to do it now, because there was no guarantee as to what shape I would be in after surgery.

Ever prepared, I added a new command to Harry's vocabulary—"Owww." The core biopsy two years ago had been a breeze until Harry body-slammed my breast with the full force of his 75-pound puppy frame. My breast turned a rainbow of blues, purples, and blacks. It hurt. Not wanting to take any chances with the upcoming surgery, I spent a few minutes each day training him to sit and stay if I said, "Owww."

Lymphedema. The word alone was enough to start me hyperventilating. The surgeon would do a sentinel node biopsy on my right breast, but if the node was positive he would remove all the lymph nodes, setting me up for the potential of lymphedema. How would I cope with limited use of my right arm? Shopping would be a problem if I couldn't heft a 40-pound bag of dog food. While doing household chores, I watched to see what I was going to have to farm out. I knew I would need help, and I hated having to ask for it.

So, for the first time in my life, I asked for help and the response stunned me. A neighbor volunteered to do grocery shopping. Just in case, I computerized our regular grocery list and then sorted it by aisle so she could get in and out quickly.

A friend volunteered to be housekeeper. I tidied the house, to make it easier to clean. Other friends offered food and to drive me to chemo if the need arose. It brought me to tears, every time I thought about the offers of help and the number of times friends and family said, "I love you."

All too quickly, the time before surgery passed and suddenly it was the night before. My surgery was scheduled for 2:00 p.m. on September 3—five years and one day to the day my father had died.

By now, my anxiety had channeled into "what ifs?" Ever prepared, I keyed in a one-page list of instructions for my friend Abby, who would wait with Sam during the surgery and then stay with me in the hospital. My cousin Amy was coming from Alabama and would stay until the surgery was over.

The years of experience in information processing showed in my list. It was a decision tree of "if-then" statements. If the surgery goes well, stop here. If the surgery doesn't go well, call Sam's brother—he can be here in three hours, then call my shrink—here's her emergency number, here's the phone number of a friend who is also a shrink if you can't get my shrink, and by the way, here's a bottle of tranquilizers for Sam, if it's real bad.

"Take care of Sam, first. He's got to take care of me. I like to think the doctors will be looking after me," I told Abby as we talked one last time that night. "I left a twenty-dollar bill, so once surgery starts, go feed him. I've packed a kit bag for him—munchies and bottled water, but he'll need to eat. I'm leaving you my cell phone to make calls. Also, promise me you won't tell anybody if I wake up screaming in the recovery room, 'Put 'em back on!'"

There was one more thing left on my list that only Sam and I could do. Although reconstruction was out for the time being, I wanted to document my breasts. That way, down the road, if I wanted reconstruction, a plastic surgeon could see what the originals looked like.

I slipped my shirt off and Sam took pictures. Pictures from all angles—front, side, three-quarter profile. Grabbing a yardstick and standing with my back flat against the bathroom wall, we measured my D-cup breasts, both in a bra and without. From my back to my nipple was exactly twelve inches.

"I love your breasts," Sam said, hugging me when we finished. "But I love *you* so much more."

The next morning, the nurse handed me a pen. I opened my hospital gown and wrote "yes" on both breasts, careful not to come near the mark made earlier that would guide the surgeon to the sentinel lymph node. I remembered writing "no" on my mother's right breast seven years earlier. They couldn't make a mistake with me. I was going to lose both breasts. I was tempted to draw smiley frowns. I said goodbye to my breasts.

A few minutes later, as I climbed on the operating table, I prayed for strength. When the anesthesiologist injected something into my IV line, I closed my eyes. My last conscious thought was: it all does end in the blink of an eye.

They tell me I woke up in the recovery room wailing, "Nodes?" "No nodes," was the response. The wonder drug I'd been given didn't just mask pain but made you forget it. "Nodes?" I couldn't remember from one second to the next. "No nodes?" It finally registered. The sentinel node biopsy had shown my lymph nodes were clean.

After post-op, I went to a private room on the extended recovery floor. Once settled, Sam, Amy, and Abby gathered around me. We held hands and prayed a prayer of thanksgiving. Thanks for the cancer not being in the lymph nodes, and thanks for me making it through surgery without major mishap.

Amy left to go back to Alabama, then I sent Sam home to check on Harry and get some rest. Abby would spend the night with me in the hospital. The surgery was over and the drugs were wearing off. I was tired and hungry, having been without food or water for almost twenty hours. The nurse who had helped settle me in my room, refused to give me anything but water, citing concerns about my history of nausea after surgery.

"Look, I'm not nauseous," I insisted. "I'm hungry."

"We've got some gelatin. Let's see if you keep that down," she said, slapping a blood pressure cuff on my left arm. "Your blood pressure is down. We need to get you up and walking."

"My blood pressure is always down after I have surgery. It is always on the low side of normal anyway. Check the pre-op assessment—my pressure was 90/70. If I get moving, then can I have something to eat?"

"We'll see," she replied, ignoring what I had said.

Abby on one side, nurse on the other, I gingerly got up out of the hospital bed without using my arms. I was heavily bandaged around the chest and the tape was constricting. I had two drains—one for each breast. Made of semi-transparent plastic and egg-shaped, they were clipped to my hospital gown. I examined the fluid collecting in them. Wincing, I tried to move my arms. It hurt less than I would have thought, but I didn't have much range of movement. I stood up and walked to the bathroom. Then I wolfed down the sugar-free lime gelatin, and I was still starving.

I asked for more food, only to be told that "food service" is closed. They had bouillon, if I wanted it.

"I want real food," I told Abby after Nurse Ratchet left the room. "Go hit the food court for me. I'll take whatever is quickest."

While she was gone, I tried flexing my arms. It wasn't bad. Tentatively, I tried to raise both arms at the shoulders. It was tight, but not a lot of pain. So far no pain medication since post-op.

Before I knew it, Abby was back. "The only place open had burgers so I got you two cheeseburgers and some fries."

I ate it all and loved every morsel. I couldn't remember the last time I had had burgers and fries. It was heaven.

The nursing shift changed, and the new nurse harped on my low pressure. "If your blood pressure isn't up, you can't go home tomorrow. Your temperature is up a little, too. You need to get moving."

"Okay, that does it. Tell me how many laps I need to do around the nurses' station. I want to go home tomorrow."

"You just need to walk," she said on the way out of the room.

I thought of my mother. Years ago, in the days of Medicare's drive-by mastectomies covering only a twenty-four-hour stay, I had argued with her surgeon before surgery. The surgeon had told me bluntly that if my mother needed to stay longer in the hospital, she'd find a way to keep her there.

But my mother had her own ideas. Seventy-nine years old, crippled with arthritis and having survived four heart attacks, she'd gone home barely twenty-four hours after her mastectomy. If she could do it, so would I.

I said to Abby, "Help me get up. Then follow me, in case I fall." I moved slowly and had trouble with the IV pole. My arms didn't swing and sometimes the tape pulled on the bandage on my chest, but I completed a lap around the nurses' station, Abby at my side pushing the IV pole. As we moved toward my room, I made a point of turning and baring my teeth at Nurse Ratchet, who sat at the nurses' station. I was less than four hours out of the recovery room.

"Your blood pressure's low. We need to get you walking," a nursing assistant said after waking me at 1:00 a.m. This guy was new, I hadn't seen him before.

"I've been walking. Talk to my nurse." I turned my head to go back to sleep. Abby and I had made hourly laps around the nurses' station, and for good measure, just before turning in at midnight, we did *two* laps. It was getting easier for me to move. There was surprisingly little pain. I hadn't had any pain medication since post-op. I was tired and had fallen asleep on my own. I yawned.

He was back. "I talked to your nurse and she said you've been walking. I'll check you again at 8:00 a.m.," he said.

When he left, I turned to Abby. "Screw it. That was the first time I'd gotten to sleep. If they're so worried about my low blood pressure then we're gonna raise it before eight o'clock. What time does the food court open?"

"I think six thirty."

"Be there when it opens and get me three big cups of coffee. The caffeine will boost my blood pressure. I'm going to go home tomorrow, even if I have to sign myself out against doctor's orders."

After drinking three large cups of coffee, the caffeine worked like a charm. My blood pressure was up. At nine o'clock the next morning I was free to go home.

Home never looked so good. Harry sniffed me up one side and down the other when I walked in. I plopped down in my favorite easy chair in the den and winced as I felt a drain pull.

The drains were a hassle. We were told we had to empty them twice a day and chart the amount of fluid output, which would determine when the drains came out. I pinned the drains to my pajama tops, but their ends poked if I tried to roll on my side. I would have to sleep on my back.

We checked my temperature several times during the day, because I couldn't tell if I had a hot flash or a fever. It was always normal. We had a blood pressure cuff, and took my blood pressure twice—once right after I came home and once before bed. It was right at my baseline, normal for me.

The first night I tried sleeping upstairs in our bed, but the pillows to keep my arms elevated kept sliding. And then there was the cat problem. When I sprawled in bed, Arthur crawled up to snuggle, sniffed my left drain, then swiped at it.

I finally decided to sleep in my favorite easy chair in the den. Considered a chair and a half, it was comfortable and I had fallen asleep many a night there in front of the television. I padded the arms with pillows, because I was warned to keep my arms elevated, and slept soundly. Harry slept on the floor beside my chair.

That chair became my headquarters. I sprawled in it to read, and

I forced myself to stretch my arms periodically. My favorite posture for watching television was with my fingers laced and my arms over my head. The first time I tried that, I was tight, but soon it became easier. I forced myself to stretch my arms out to my sides, as far as the bandages would allow. Time and time again, I was amazed at the absence of pain.

Three days after surgery, I couldn't resist peeling back the edge of a bandage for a peek at where my right breast had been. My breast was replaced by a long row of silver, surgical staples. It looked exactly like a zipper.

I sniffed as I pushed the bandage back in place. No deodorant and I was ripe. I had not had a shower or bath since the morning before my surgery. My hair was so oily even the cats were trying to clean it.

I healed and passed the days. I was so grateful just to be alive that, for the time being, the loss of my breasts seemed insignificant. I had jumped one hurdle in this race—surgery. The next would come with the pathology results.

A week after surgery and it was time for the drains to come out. I felt like a caged animal that had finally been freed. I had not wanted to leave the house until the drains were gone. I threw a shirt on over my T-shirt and drove myself to the doctor's office. Sam followed me there so he could go on to work.

It took just seconds for the surgeon to remove the drains, and I didn't feel a thing. We talked while he was doing it. It would still be a few more days before the final pathology would be in, but he explained the preliminary report.

He told me it was good. The infiltrating tumor in the right breast was only 1.2 centimeters (about the size of a dime) with no sign of vascular or lymphatic involvement, encircled by fibrosis—my body had started to wall it off with scar tissue.

The most frightening part of the pathology was the left breast.

One phrase leapt out at me from the report: "A 2.3 centimeter by 1.8 centimeter by 1.8 ill-defined mass. . . . The mass shows finger-like projections." Finger-like projections—tentacles holding an area about the size of a quarter. I shuddered, thinking DCIS had been reaching out to grasp the entire breast.

Walking out of the doctor's office, I decided to own my flatness. If traffic wasn't bad, I could just make the breast-cancer support group meeting at The Wellness Community. I was interested in seeing what other women thought.

"Am I flat or what?" I said as I walked into the meeting room.

"You look great," said the facilitator.

"How long has it been?" asked one of the women.

"A week," I said proudly.

"Lookin' good," said another.

"Nodes?" one woman questioned.

"No nodes," I said.

"Go, girl!" two women said in unison, as we made high-fives.

"You know, I think this is the first time I've seen the top of my stomach since puberty," I said, looking down and laughing.

They all laughed with me. Then one by one they offered their support and encouragement, knowing I was waiting for the final pathology report. The group was emotionally validating. It was safe. These women were further ahead of me in this race and had clocked many laps. I had only jumped the first hurdle: surgery. The next hurdle would come with the final pathology—the question of chemotherapy.

After the support group meeting, I decided to go shopping. I knew I would need a new, more sensitive razor to shave under my arms. Already, I could see the progression from Frenchwoman to hairy ape. Soon the hair under my arms would be long enough to braid. It was starting to itch.

In the local discount store I pondered the dozens of safety razors.

I looked up when a woman bumped my cart and, as usual, I glanced at her chest. Well-dressed, in her early forties, she was flat like me. Maybe even flatter. Her eyes went to my chest then caught mine. She smiled and nodded before moving away. Sisterhood.

A week later, the final pathology report was in, and bleary-eyed at 8:00 a.m., Sam and I sat waiting in the oncologist's office.

"How are you healing?" the oncologist asked as she strode into the room.

"I'm good. So what's the verdict? Do I need chemo?" I took a deep breath.

"No," she said, smiling, looking very pleased. "We caught this early enough. It was a small tumor, slow growing, and highly hormone receptive. I want to put you on tamoxifen for five years."

"I'll do it," I said, thrilled. In my mind I sailed over a major hurdle.

*   *   *   *   *

So, what is it like losing your breasts? It was the unspoken question from friends and family. It's not uncomfortable, though it feels like my body's center of gravity has shifted. My posture has changed, but not to the shoulders-hunched-in "protective" posture that I had expected. I keep trying to tuck my pelvis under to compensate for the shift but those muscles won't cooperate. With or without prostheses, weighted or not, I think I stand straighter. I have to, and I make a conscious effort to monitor my posture, taking every opportunity to catch my reflection in a mirror. I refuse to become the Hunchback of Notre Dame.

The first time I wore a pair of prostheses, it was the five-dollar soft guys that were filled with something akin to pillow stuffing. Very poofy, very soft, and very light. Ten days after my surgery Harry needed to go to the vet. Two years old and 100-plus pounds, he was mostly trained to the "Owww" command, but I cringed at the thought of what a body-slam would do to my tender chest. I wore the mastectomy camisole I had bought prior to surgery. It was larger than a traditional camisole and had pockets at the bust line. I was surprised at the sense of protection I felt.

Before surgery, I had bought a mastectomy bra and a weighted inexpensive pair of swimmer's B-cup prostheses. The bra's cups were seamed, not smooth like my regular bras, and it was heavily reinforced. A soft fabric was sewn to the back of the cup and would hold the prosthesis in place. It had been the best looking of the lot I had seen that day in the mastectomy boutique.

The first time I put on the bra and prostheses, I pulled on a cotton turtle neck, a staple of my fall wardrobe. Examining myself in the mirror, I decided my bust looked like something out of the 1950s—pointy breasts with bra seams showing through the cotton fabric. So not me. And what's worse, the prostheses I had bought were seamed and pointy, too. Their seams came together in the center of the prostheses to form a totally unnatural looking pseudo-erect nipple. Think June Cleaver with erect nipples wearing a tight sweater. Or today, Madonna in a cone bra. But I had bought the pointy guys so I was stuck with them—no returns on prostheses. I would have to make do until I could get a proper pair. Pointy nipples and all, I headed off to the nearest fabric shop. A little soft padding and a cover would work for the time being.

I had my sewing basket out and was working on a prosthesis when Sam came home that evening.

"Ah, my industrious little wife, " he chuckled, bending down to kiss me. "Some women do needlepoint, you make boobs." He eyed the prosthesis and plopped down his laptop.

I wasn't shy about letting Sam see my incision scars; in fact, we made a point of checking them periodically in the beginning. The surgeon had been proud of his work—the scars were perfectly symmetrical. My battle scars. Of course, the scars are numb, just like the area under my right arm where the surgeon removed the sentinel node. Nerves were severed and may not grow back.

There's a long mirror in the foyer at the foot of the stairs in our house. Every time I go up or down the steps, I make a point of glancing in it. I check to see if I am hunched over and then correct my posture. The more time that passes since the surgery, the easier it is to maintain a good posture. There's a mirror in the antique sideboard in the kitchen, and I check my reflection there. Are the prostheses riding "high," up near my shoulders, or at an appropriate height?

The only problem has been the bras. I keep reminding myself that I had to experiment to find comfortable bras before the surgery. It's no different now. Problem is I can't tell if a bra works until I've worn it for a day or two, so returns are impossible. After spending fifty dollars for a "seamless, smooth cup" mastectomy bra that was miserably uncomfortable and rode up, I have forsworn mastectomy bras.

I have made an art of studying bras. I have found some that I like and that go with a new pair of prostheses. Rounder, softer, more natural. I'm comfortable.

*   *   *   *   *

It's now been several months since my surgery, and I have no regrets about my choice. It may seem odd, but I'm thankful for everything that has happened and especially for the women I've met. Breast cancer creates a powerful bond. I still tear up when I think of all the women who opened their hearts and their shirts to me, as I made a difficult decision.

I heard from one of my cousins recently who had a blip on her mammogram and was worried. She's scheduled for another mam-

mogram and an ultrasound. I hope her doctor is just being hyper-
vigilant because of my diagnosis. But if this turns out to be breast
cancer, I envision myself offering her a hand at the starting line of
the race, as so many women did for me. Side by side we'll run her
first lap together, keeping our eyes on the prize.

*Not long after Selden's bilateral mastectomy, she learned that she
needed a hysterectomy. Fortunately, her results were benign and she has
made a full recovery. Selden has no desire to pursue breast reconstruction.*

Robin McILvain

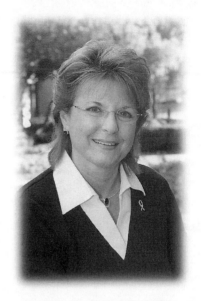

was born in Cincinnati, Ohio. As a young girl, she and her family lived in Libya and Morocco for several years, until the sudden death of her mother. Returning to Cincinnati, Robin later married her high school sweetheart to whom she has been happily married for thirty-seven years. She and her husband raised a son and daughter and now are doting grandparents to three young grandchildren. Despite lifelong health problems, Robin continued to work in various management positions in sales and construction, and became a licensed real estate agent. Robin is an avid reader and also enjoys scrapbooking (at her daughter's encouragement) to chronicle family events. Drawing from her own life experiences, along with her strong sense of spirituality, she finds purpose and fulfillment inspiring others who seek her advice. An active participant in her breast-cancer support group at The Wellness Community in Atlanta, Robin helps newly diagnosed patients through their battle with breast cancer.

DIAGNOSIS PROFILE

Age at diagnosis:	50 years old
Family history:	No knowledge
Symptoms:	None—abnormal mammogram
Surgery:	Stereotactic core biopsy
	Lumpectomy
Biopsy results:	Ductal carcinoma in situ (DCIS)
	Comedo with necrosis & focal spread to lobules
	Stage: 0
	Tumor size: 1.4 cm.
	Nodes: none removed
	Grade: 3
Radiation therapy:	28 treatments
Hormonal therapy:	Tamoxifen recommended
Pre-diagnosis:	11 years of HRT
Complications:	Lymphedema

If I were a horse, I would have been shot a long time ago!

Happy Fiftieth Birthday . . . You Have Breast Cancer!

ROBIN McILVAIN

As I approached my fiftieth year, I eagerly looked forward to beginning the next half-century of my life's journey. Up to that point, I had faced far too many challenges, including complex health-related ones. Now, as my birthday neared, I was filled with excitement and gratitude—not only had I reached this wonderful milestone, but I was also beginning a new career in residential real estate. For health reasons, I had left a very stressful job the year before and decided, after serious reflection, to head in a new direction. I wanted to be my own boss, work independently, create my own opportunities, and focus on taking better care of my fragile health.

By the time I was in my late forties, I had been hospitalized more than twenty times to surgically remove, repair, or explore some part of my body. If I were a horse, I would have been shot a long time ago! Despite precarious health and my numerous medical conditions, I never expected to hear a diagnosis of breast cancer. I had no knowledge of it in my family, though I now know that a majority of women diagnosed do not have a family history of it. Interestingly enough, only 5 to 10 percent of all breast cancer is actually hereditary and can come from either the paternal or maternal side, if not from both. With my medical history being so complex, I believed surely I would be spared a diagnosis of cancer—any cancer! Upon reading risk factors for breast cancer, I related only to one of them: I began menstruating at the age of eleven. I attributed this early onset of my period to the emotional trauma that occurred the day after my eleventh birthday—my mother was killed in a car accident. Her untimely death was devastating and brought much pain and change within my family. When I was thirty-two, I had a hysterectomy, which brought an early end to my periods, making the risk factor for cancer even less significant.

Over the years, I diligently had annual mammograms and breast exams as part of my overall disease prevention program. Six years after my hysterectomy, I chose to take hormonal replacement therapy because I started having uncomfortable menopausal symptoms—I still had one ovary. A few years later, I was switched to estrogen without progesterone when studies found it unnecessary for women without a uterus to take both. I asked my gynecologist how long I should be on it and he asked, "How long do you plan on living?"

"At least until I'm a hundred years old."

"Then you can stop at ninety-nine!" he said.

Just a few months before my breast-cancer diagnosis, I had decided to switch from a conventional synthetic brand to a more natural phytoestrogen product (Remifemin). Over the years, doctors had encouraged me to stay on estrogen, hoping it would protect my heart and bones—it didn't. Like other members of my family, I am challenged with coronary artery disease. I also have severe osteoporosis. Who would have thought I would be told to discontinue all estrogen forty-nine years short of my target date?

On the fateful day that my annual mammogram showed an abnormality, nothing unusual had happened at my appointment to alert me that anything was wrong, so when the films were developed, I left. Looking back, I remember reading the daily quote on my calendar that morning: "I love my past, I love my present. I'm not ashamed of what I've had, and I'm not sad because I have it no longer."—Colette. Underneath was written: "Acceptance of our life just as it is and as it has been opens many more doors to the future than fighting with it does." Prophetic words as I opened the mail on New Year's Eve day, a little over a week after my mammogram and the day before my fiftieth birthday.

As my husband, David, waited in the car for me—we were on our way to our daughter Christy's house to celebrate our granddaughter Kelsey's second birthday—I quickly glanced through the mail, setting aside my birthday cards to open the next day. I noticed the envelope from The Women's Center where I had my mammograms, and it took a moment to register what it contained. Then remembering, I opened it, thinking I was all set for another year. In disbelief, I read, "an area in recent bilateral mammogram needs further evaluation." What did that mean? I was instructed to contact my doctor for a more detailed report, but the long holiday weekend had started. My heart sank as I read it again. From somewhere deep inside, I felt like screaming at the top of my lungs: *No! Please no, not now . . . not ever! There has already been too much!*

I suddenly remembered my husband waiting in the car and wondered how I could tell him, or maybe I should wait until I knew more. Leaving the letter on the counter, I went out to the car with an initial decision to say nothing—just yet. Throughout our marriage, we had survived many challenges, including my ongoing health problems. When David saw the look on my face and asked if I was okay, I knew I could not keep this from him. Hesitantly, I told him of the letter and my "gut feeling" about its outcome, and of the overpowering urge to scream, an urge that I was suppressing so as not to lose control. His immediate reaction was to turn around and go home, but I knew that celebrating our granddaughter's birthday would be a welcome distraction, so I encouraged him to continue driving. He reluctantly agreed.

We were silent the remainder of the ride, deep in our own thoughts. I hoped my gut feeling was wrong, and I prayed for courage and strength. Mary Tyler Moore once said in an interview: "Pain nourishes courage. You can't be brave if you've only had wonderful things happen to you."

Soon after we arrived, Christy noticed I was unusually quiet. Because of our special relationship, I knew she would want to know, and we went into another room to talk. Sharing my news with her was extremely difficult as I fought back the tears. Although my children grew up watching me overcome one malady after another, I was always the eternal optimist, the strong one who reassured others that I would soon be well enough to jump back into my very busy life. Showing vulnerability versus strength was uncomfortable. Then, a gripping fear hit me. If I were diagnosed with breast cancer, how would that affect the future odds for my daughter, granddaughter, and sisters? Would we now have our own family history of this disease? I hugged her tightly as we both cried and tried to sound convincing that all would turn out well.

That night, David and I went to see the film *Stepmom*, starring Julia Roberts. Not a good choice for two reasons. First, it was about a mother dying of cancer. Second, the daughter in the film was about the same age as I had been when I lost my mother. With the anniversary of her death two days away, I cried through the movie.

The next morning, on my fiftieth birthday, I lay in bed and thought about the fact that I was one of millions of other baby boomers who was a half-century old. A quote that always reassures me of a long life came to mind: *God put me on earth to accomplish a certain number of things; right now I am so far behind, I will never die.*

As I dressed that day, I looked at my breasts in the mirror, wondering which one needed "further evaluation," since the letter had not specified. Intuitively, I felt it was my right one, having had most of my medical problems on that side of my body. Before a recent Christmas party, I had a jacket altered (it was a little snug) by an Asian woman who commented that Asian women had very small breasts and complained about hers. I offered some of mine, saying it would eliminate the need to alter my jacket. We laughed that women are never satisfied with their bodies. Looking in the mirror two weeks later, I told God I was only kidding when I had complained of my breast size!

The long holiday weekend finally ended, and before I could follow up on the letter, I took my husband to the airport for his annual two-week business trip to Asia. Under the circumstances, it was a difficult parting. A message from my gynecologist's nurse was waiting for me when I got back home asking me to call about the results of my recent mammogram. Before returning the call, I phoned The Women's Center and learned that it would be three weeks before I could get in for a re-check appointment. Nothing I said could get me in sooner. I was told that my doctor's office could call on my behalf and an appointment could become "available" within forty-eight hours! Frustrated, I called my gynecologist's office for help. Then, my husband telephoned to say his connecting flight was cancelled due to weather conditions, and I returned to the airport to pick him up, happy to have him home for two more days.

My mammogram results from my gynecologist were waiting on my fax machine when I got back from the airport. I was right. The abnormality was in my right breast. There were calcifications that could possibly be hiding a lesion, requiring further evaluation. I had to put the report aside and my thoughts with it in order to spend the rest of the day and evening preparing and presenting my first real estate contract. Thankfully, it went well, and I fell into bed later that night, exhausted.

It took several more frustrating attempts to get a sooner-than-later re-check appointment. Two days later, I was "squeezed in" at The Women's Center thanks to my gynecologist's nurse. She was successful in moving up my appointment, but was told to tell me that they did not consider my re-check an emergency. "If a mammogram is abnormal and suspicious for breast cancer, what would constitute an emergency?" I asked. She had no answer.

Between my new real estate career, and health and family issues, I didn't have a whole lot of time to dwell on any one thing. Feeling my stamina waning, I pushed myself with my usual denial of mind over body and had ongoing conversations with God. During the wee hours of the morning when sleep escaped me, I e-mailed friends. They allowed me to express anger for the lack of control I felt over my body—this was something that my "type A" personality could not "fix." In *Webster's New World Dictionary* the word *accept* is defined "to receive willingly." Having a fighting spirit and deep faith and being raised in a generation influenced by clichés such as "no pain, no gain," "mind over body," and "use it or lose it," I continually pushed myself. Over the years, I learned to follow healthy lifestyle choices with diet, vitamin supplementation, weight control, and exercise. So, why wasn't it working for me? One of my doctors told me to think about where I would be otherwise!

The day before my re-check appointment, my husband left on his business trip and was soon halfway around the world—neither of us slept that night. I left early the next morning—my appointment was for 7:45 a.m., and after sitting for an hour, I finally heard the mammography technician call my name. She tried to reassure me that these re-checks turned out just fine most of the time. She explained that the newer mammography machines were more sensitive in picking up powder specks or deodorant on the skin, which was the case in a high percentage of need for re-checks. As my breast was positioned in the machine, she said she would take several magnified views to get a better look at the area in question. After the films were developed, she showed me the calcifications that were covering an area beyond the scope of the X-ray equipment. She went to show them to the radiologist while I waited nervously in the room. When she returned, and with my stomach now in knots, I asked if I could get the results that day. Out she went again to speak to the radiologist. He offered to see me, but said he was very busy and could only spend a couple of minutes with me. I was grateful for even that time. I was shown the "cluster of calcifications" in the outer portion of my right breast that was not present in previous mammograms. They looked like very small dots, as if someone had taken the point of a pen and poked the film multiple times. It was hard to believe they could represent cancer, but what did I know? It was abnormal and the radiologist recommended a biopsy. He assured me that there was a good chance this would be a benign condition; it was in most cases.

As I walked to my car, I tried to sort out what I had just heard. After all the years of normal mammograms, why was it I now needed a biopsy? I always had symptoms when something was wrong. How could there be a problem with no symptoms? Driving home, I tried to ignore my gut feelings on the outcome of the biopsy.

My gynecologist's nurse had given me the name of a breast surgeon, Dr. I., someone she highly recommended, and I made an appointment with him for the following week. Then some good news came. Negotiations for my first real estate contract were successful, and I planned to stay focused for my clients until their transaction closed. There was also a happy visit from my dear friend

Sandy, who lived out of state. We had shared a very special friend-ship for more than twenty years. With David still out of the country on business, it was comforting to have Sandy with me.

The morning of my appointment with Dr. I., Marion, another longtime friend, who lives nearby, called and said she wanted to go with me. A fifteen-year breast-cancer survivor herself (Marion also shares her story in this book), she knew exactly how I was feeling. But since this was only a consultation visit, I assured her I would be fine. As I hung up the phone, intuitively I knew she did not accept my going alone. Sure enough, I was right. At the doctor's office, as I was signing in, I heard a voice say, "Robin, you're late." I turned around and there she was. I was grateful for her presence, especially since I waited for over an hour to be seen. Marion accompanied me to an examining room, and a few minutes later I met Dr. I. I didn't doubt his professional experience and expertise, but I was disap-pointed by his bedside manner, or lack thereof, and the disrespect he showed from the moment he came into the room. He seemed rushed and abrupt, as well as uninterested in anything I said.

He quickly reviewed my mammogram films, spoke to his nurse as if Marion and I were invisible, then gave me his expert opinion. He thought there was a 20 percent chance that what he saw on my mammogram was malignant. I told him I prayed he was correct. He said he would do a "stereotactic core biopsy" and asked how soon I wanted it done. As soon as possible was my answer. I told him what I had read on the Internet about this type of biopsy. He was instantly critical of patients obtaining information via the Internet, saying there was a lot of inaccurate information out there. When I explained what I had read, he admitted my information about the procedure was correct. I told him of sites on the Internet that I had visited and that I believed in being a proactive patient who wanted to empower herself to learn as much as possible. When I said I wanted to "partner with my doctors in my care," he nodded halfheartedly, left to check his schedule, and returned to tell me the biopsy could be done the next morning. I was relieved, but still felt this "guru" of breast surgeons (as my gynecologist's nurse called him) was arrogant and lacked compassion. This time when Marion insisted on bringing me back the next day, I did not try to dissuade her. Unfortunately, that evening she phoned to say that she had to leave town immediately due to a family emergency. She hated that she would not be able to go with me, but I tried to assure her I would be okay, saying this was not my first medical procedure, and I just wanted to get it behind me.

Unfortunately, nothing I had read about a stereotactic core biopsy prepared me for my experience the next day. A nurse led me to the procedure room, where I saw a table with a large hole in it, just as it had looked on the Internet. She handed me a small paper gown and told me to undress from the waist up with the gown opened in the front, and she would be back. When she returned, she instructed me to lie on the table face down with my right breast in the large hole, and that no matter what happened during the procedure, I was not to move once Dr. I. began. Lying face down on the table, she positioned my right breast and said Dr. I. would arrive in a few minutes. The nurse and I made small talk for a while, then she had to leave the room.

When Dr. I. finally arrived, I had waited for over an hour. Again, he acted rushed. He offered no explanation until I said that my biopsy was scheduled an hour ago. He said he had another biopsy before mine and offered no apology. "Lie perfectly still," he said, and I obeyed. But given what followed, I had no idea how difficult that would be. I felt the injection go into my breast to numb it. Later, he said that the cut in my breast was made before I was given any numbing medication. Thankfully, I had not felt that. What I did feel was an excruciating, burning sensation that seared through my breast from what felt like a stapler gun going into it. I cried out in pain, with tears welling up in my eyes, when Dr. I. lashed out at me for moving and announced he would not continue. My head, as instructed, was turned away from him, and his nurse sat beside me. With a sympathetic look, she quietly asked if I could continue. I knew if I did not allow him to proceed, it would delay a diagnosis. I asked for more numbing medication, which I got, and after waiting a few more minutes to make sure my breast was numb, he began again. This time, the pain was bearable.

Afterward, while the doctor bandaged the cut in my breast, I learned he removed more than a dozen tissue samples, saying it was more than he usually took. With confidence, he now predicted I had only a 10 percent risk of cancer. He quickly added that if the results were benign, it was still an "abnormal" finding, and I should definitely have a follow-up mammogram in six months.

"What if it's not benign?" I asked.

"Let's not go there because it would take an hour to discuss," he replied. When he said to call him in a week for the results, I questioned having to wait an entire week.

"That's how long it takes the lab," he said brusquely. I was told his nurse would give me the results if benign; if they weren't, I would be speaking to him. Before leaving, I said I would rely on his expertise, as well as his optimism that my results would be benign. I had little faith in the latter.

Waiting for the results became one of the longest weeks of my life. Several nights, I awoke hearing, "Oh my God, it's cancer" coming out of my mouth. Never before with any other health problem had this happened, even though there had been potential cancer diagnoses for my colon, thyroid, and ovary. Was I being warned? Prepared? No matter how busy I tried to keep myself, the days crept by, and I had to keep reminding myself to "breathe."

David returned home, tired, jet-lagged and sick, the day before I got the biopsy results. We were both happy that he was home. I shared the good news that the CAT scan of my liver was normal (yes, liver problems had necessitated this test, which was done on the same day I first met with Dr. I.), but another diagnostic procedure to find the problem was suggested, pending the breast biopsy report. Then I happily reported that Christy was expecting our second grandchild. That night I slept little, but was grateful that I had made it through the week. The phone calls, e-mails, and cards from family and friends had comforted me. I hoped the prayers being said for me would be answered.

To calm me before calling Dr. I., I began the next day by listening to a meditation tape by Carolyn Myss, author of the book *Why People Don't Heal and How They Can*. For the past week, as I listened to her morning and evening tapes, they helped "center" me. When the tape ended, I put on the coffee and decided to call mid-morning, hoping David would be awake by then. Before I knew it, it was time to call and my heart started to race. I was relieved to connect to his nurse right away. When asked to hold on while she pulled my file, I held my breath. It seemed to take forever before she came back on the line. I heard the rustling of papers and then she said she needed to go over several files with Dr. I., but he was in surgery and would call me back between 11:30 a.m. and 1:30 p.m. As I hung up the phone, my stomach knotted and my heart continued to race. I remembered that Dr. I. had said that I would talk to him if the results were not benign. At that moment, I knew the results and could no longer deny the gut feeling I'd had from the day I received my initial mammography results in the mail. I replayed my conversation with the nurse, trying to find something positive in it, when the phone rang. On the other end was my friend Rhonda, asking about my results in her caring voice. I told her I was still waiting, but was, of course, thinking the worst. We spent the rest of the morning on the phone, which helped to pass the time until the doctor called. The phone rang at 1:30 p.m. I thought my heart would give out.

Dr. I. said the biopsy showed cancer cells in all the tissue samples he had removed. He then surprised me by saying, "But you already knew, didn't you?" Although my mouth suddenly felt as dry as the Mojave Desert, I managed to blurt out that I had prayed very hard to be wrong.

Then, as if he were thinking out loud, he said, "I'll do a lumpectomy and remove lymph nodes." He countered that with, "No, I won't remove any nodes." He became very clinical and I tried to keep up with what he was saying, but it was extremely difficult to concentrate on the rest of the conversation. I was still reeling from the words *there were cancer cells*. I asked for a time frame to have the lumpectomy, considering my ongoing liver problem, and was told not to wait any longer than thirty days. He emphatically said to call him as soon as I found out from my gastroenterologist if I was at risk to have this surgery. Again, as though thinking out loud, he said he would schedule the operation while awaiting my call.

I was paralyzed in my chair as I hung up the phone. And devastated. "Happy fiftieth birthday, Robin . . . you have breast cancer!" I said to myself. It was not even a month since I'd turned fifty, and "ductal carcinoma in situ" (DCIS) was one of my birthday presents!

David was leaving the next day on a business trip. I slowly got up to go to him, taking a deep breath, but starting to cry. In the safety of his arms, I heard myself say, "I'm not sure I have the strength or will to fight another disease. I'm so tired of battling health problems."

With worry and concern in his voice, David said quietly, "You have to keep fighting." Holding me tight, I knew he was right. I was a survivor and somehow, by the grace of God, I would survive this.

After a good cry, I spent the remainder of the day on the phone. In between phone calls from family and friends wanting to know my biopsy results, I left messages for my gynecologist and gastroenterologist. I told Dr. D., my gynecologist, about my awful experience with Dr. I., the surgeon that his nurse had so highly recommended. He offered to refer me to another surgeon, if after the weekend, I decided to make the change. As I hung up the phone, I knew I would call him on Monday. For now, I would try to get through the weekend . . . one minute at a time.

All my past surgeons had been men, so when Dr. D. recommended a female doctor, I told him this would be a new experience for me. He was very hopeful I would like her.

Although on the appointment day I had to wait for more than an hour, when I finally met with the surgeon, Dr. S., I liked her instantly. She put me completely at ease with her caring manner—I knew I was in good hands. I told her about my experience with Dr. I. and that I wanted a second opinion. After looking at my films and reports, she explained that my particular form of breast cancer, up until two years before, had always been treated by surgical removal of the entire breast, a mastectomy. But with the newer mammography machines, microcalcifications are detected sooner, making diagnosis and treatment easier. However, this form of breast cancer was still considered tricky surgery since it can neither be felt nor seen, except by mammography. She said she was hopeful she could remove enough of it and that radiation therapy should "clean up" any leftover cells. She also said most breast surgeons were currently recommending lumpectomy with radiation therapy for DCIS and were obtaining the same results as a mastectomy. At that moment, it was important to me to keep both my breasts.

Like Dr. I., she did not plan on removing lymph nodes but would take out enough breast tissue to get "clean margins" with no cancer cells in the surrounding tissue of the tumor mass, thus eliminating additional surgery. On my mammogram she, too, pointed out the calcifications extending to the outer portion of my breast and the film's edge, making it difficult to know how extensive an area they covered. By the end of my visit, it was too late to schedule my operation. Since it was Friday, I was told to call her office on Monday. A long and tiring day was over, but at least, for the first time, I felt I was being treated with compassion by a doctor who had my fragile health in her hands.

On the day of my operation, I had to be at the hospital by 5:30 a.m. The only good thing about that ungodly hour was no rush-hour traffic. When David and I arrived (he was home for a change), I was taken to the radiology department to have a very thin metal wire inserted into my breast through a needle that would outline the area of calcifications that would be removed. The procedure began as another unpleasant and painful one, until I asked the radiologist to administer more numbing medication. Once he made sure I was numb enough, the rest of the procedure was uneventful, and I felt nothing, even when a follow-up mammogram showed the wire needed adjusting.

I was taken to the pre-op area and within minutes I was in the operating room. Just before I was put to sleep, Dr. S. came and stood beside me. She took my hand and as she held it in hers, she promised to take very good care of me. Looking into her eyes, I did not doubt her for a moment, and I drifted off to sleep.

The operation went well, just as my surgeon had promised, and after a short time in recovery I was on my way home. The nurses were wonderful and had taken good care of me. Later, David told me that right after the operation, Dr. S. came to talk to him. There in the crowded waiting area, she explained what she had done to remove the cancer. She even demonstrated over her operating scrubs, using her own breast as a visual aid. Poor guy—it was too much description for him!

There is no place like home to recuperate, and it felt good being in my own bed. Initially, I found lying on my side uncomfortable, but holding a pillow between my breasts and lying on my "good side" did the trick. (I read this helpful "cushioning" suggestion in *Dr.*

Susan Love's Breast Book.) That afternoon, I enjoyed a visit with my daughter and granddaughter, and received flowers, cards, and phone calls from family and friends. I felt surrounded by so much love as I awaited my second pathology report.

Thankfully, I would not have to endure as long a wait as the first one because Dr. S. said she would have the results at my post-op visit, a few days later. At that visit she burst into the examining room with my report in hand, beaming with the news that my margins were "clean!" As she hugged me, I thanked God. She turned to David, saying, "Don't worry, she won't be dying of this cancer!" The relief he and I felt was palpable. The report stated there appeared to be no invasion of cancer cells outside the ducts into the surrounding tissue. However, the cancer cells were now described as "comedo," a type of DCIS where the cells filling the duct are more aggressive looking and have the propensity to become an invasive cancer. There was also necrosis (dead tissue). Since the first biopsy report had described the cells as non-comedo, I asked about the difference and was told they took the worst of the two when deciding treatment and prognosis. Because the histology of the tumor mass was high-grade, she recommended radiation therapy followed by five years of tamoxifen. In addition to my complex medical history, she said I now constituted a "family" history of breast cancer and hoped that by taking tamoxifen, it would prevent a recurrence in the same breast, and perhaps prevent a new cancer in the other breast, or else-where. She recommended I see a medical oncologist who would refer me to a radiation oncologist. Afterward, the oncologist would monitor me on tamoxifen over the next five years. To help the radiation team stage my treatment process, she explained there were several surgical clips in my breast outlining where the tumor mass had been. My next visit with her would be in three months when I was through with radiation therapy, and a mammogram of my right breast would be done.

During my recuperation, I began searching for a medical oncologist and was happy with the choice I made. Dr. L. and his staff could not have been kinder. After reviewing my medical history, they told me the breast cancer was not my fault—that I had done everything I could to prevent it. Following my examination, David and I spoke to Dr. L. When I asked if I could be carrying the gene that could affect my sisters, daughter, and granddaughter, he assured me that, in my case, he did not think so. He based his answer on my age and lack of breast cancer, as far as I knew, in my family history. That helped to assuage some of my guilt. He agreed with Dr. S. about taking tamoxifen. I expressed concern about taking the drug because one of its side effects is liver problems, and I did not need more liver problems! He reassured me that it would be okay to take tamoxifen, then recommended a radiation oncologist.

Dr. C. also turned out to be a caring and compassionate woman. She even told me her mother had died of breast cancer. After her death, she switched specialties in order to help other women. She explained radiation therapy and its side effects. In my case, it would exacerbate the fibromyalgia, a syndrome characterized by chronic muscle and joint pain in multiple tender points, morning stiffness, fatigue, and sleep disturbances, to name just a few symptoms of this condition. My chest wall muscle and rib cage would be affected, and she wanted me to know this before treatment began. Additionally, there would be an increase of pain in the radiated area that would never really go away. Since I have severe osteoporosis, I was concerned about rib fractures, which are also a common side effect. She assured me that with the improved radiation machines, this was no longer a problem. Since then, I have had three fractured ribs!

After the examination, she led me to the treatment room and I was introduced to the technicians. Each step was explained to me as my right breast was drawn on with a marker pen, and tape was placed over the marks. I did not get the customary permanent "tattoo" markings because of my high risk for infection. My upper body lay in a mold of warm water. The technicians called out numbers to one another as they lined me up or "staged" the daily treatment plan. Each day I would be placed into the fitted mold, maintaining the same position with my right arm raised over my head. What with the recent surgery and having fibromyalgia, it was a difficult position. I learned about daily care of my affected breast and about products, such as natural aloe, to use and what not to use. No shaving that armpit or using deodorant for the duration of treatment. Then a time was scheduled for five days a week for the next six weeks.

Right before the treatments began, as I waited for the mold that I would lie in to harden, Dr. S. called and asked me to come in for a mammogram to be absolutely sure she had removed all the calcifications. I heard myself reluctantly agree, wondering how on earth I was going to stand having a mammogram just three weeks post-op. My breast was still very tender and sore. Somehow I got through it, like I have everything else, and taking a pain pill beforehand sure helped. The technician was both sympathetic and gentle as she placed my still very tender and painful breast in the "vise" of the machine. When the films were reviewed, I was elated to hear that no more calcifications were seen. I was cleared to begin radiation.

I received news that my first real estate listing sold and the closing was in two weeks—the day after my first treatment. I then planned to take time off to complete my treatments and take care of my fragile physical and emotional well-being. I made every effort to "stay in life" by keeping in touch with family and friends and reading books that lifted my spirits. A favorite book was Sarah Ban Breathnach's *Simple Abundance*. When reading the daily passages, the words rang so true to me it was as though they were coming from my own head. Her other book, *Something More*, had the same effect. Another truly inspirational work that I believe every woman can relate to is Anne Morrow Lindbergh's *Gift from the Sea*, written back in 1955.

For most of the daily trips to and from the treatment facility, I was fortunate to have David drive me. Each treatment went quickly. In fact, it took longer to get there, put on a dressing gown, and wait my turn than to have the treatments themselves. I watched the technicians exit the room, leaving me alone to stare at the overhead machine as it went from one side to the other, emitting beams of radiation into my breast area. How safe was this radiation exposure?

Early in my treatment, I made a friend in cyberspace one night when I could not sleep. I found an Internet site where women shared their breast-cancer stories, and I e-mailed my story to one of the women. Pleasantly surprised, I received an e-mail right back from her. She wanted to know how I was doing with the radiation treatments. She seemed to understand the emotional roller coaster I was experiencing as well. We stayed in touch throughout my treatments, but once they ended, my e-mails from her did too. The ones I sent her came back "undeliverable." In retrospect, I truly believe she was a guardian angel sent to me during this difficult time—someone I could turn to in the wee hours of the morning, knowing she truly understood what I was going through. I shall never forget her and pray she is well.

Unfortunately, I experienced skin reactions from the radiation after the very first treatment. I was allergic to the tape that covered the marks on my breast. And my breast burned and itched constantly, which became a real challenge when out in public! The first time the tape was removed, it pulled layers of skin with it. With each treatment, the burning increased until the nurse gave me a tube of cream called Aquaphor to apply to the raw spots. I also used aloe lotion. Nothing helped. The springtime temperature was rising, as it often does here in the South, which caused even greater discomfort. My breast stayed on fire. The radiation oncologist looked at my skin once a week and asked how I was doing. A practical nurse who was part of the team told me how "lucky" I was to have been diagnosed via early detection with ductal carcinoma in situ, assuring me I would be fine. Without hesitating, I said that I did not feel the least bit "lucky" to have any form of breast cancer. Prevention, for me, did not mean early detection!

The side effects of radiation began to kick in—or rather, to kick me. As I grew more tired and lethargic, my skin looked worse. The tape was changed daily due to my allergic reaction. The redness and itching continued, and Dr. C. said I had one of the worst burns she'd ever seen. She asked if I would be able to continue treatment. I had one more week to go and was determined to get through it. Dr. C. recommended I take a few days off to give my skin a break. She heard no objection from me. As we talked, I told her I was beginning to second-guess my surgical choice and if I had to make it again, I would have had a mastectomy to avoid radiation. I was no stranger to radiation and its effects. Twelve years earlier, I had had radioactive iodine to my thyroid, due to Graves' disease (hyperthyroidism). It was administered internally by swallowing a radioactive capsule. What an experience that was, especially afterward, when a Geiger counter was placed at my neck. It subsequently caused problems with my salivary glands, resulting in the removal of one of them.

Although the radiation team said they could not explain the nausea I was experiencing, I found a couple of products at my local health food store that brought relief. One contained ginger root and honey (Solaray) called Ginger Trips, the other was a tasty drink (Reed's) called Raspberry Ginger Brew. Also, my decreased appetite affected my taste buds and food choices. I craved fresh carrots and tomatoes, snacked on soy bars, and drank lots of water. At the advice of my wonderful practitioner of traditional Chinese medicine, Barbara Squires, I took Siberian Ginseng for the fatigue and lethargy, along with a daily dose of vitamins.

As I headed into my last week of treatment, I fell and injured a knee. The radiation team could not believe it when I showed up on crutches, sporting a brace from thigh to ankle. I had just put away a special shoe that finally helped to heal a fractured toe, which had occurred right before my cancer diagnosis. Am I accident prone or what?!

A month after the radiation treatments, I went for my follow-up visit to Dr. C. My skin was still in pretty bad shape, but she said it would eventually heal and go from a burn to a tan and lighten over time. The swelling of my breast and underarm, along with the fatigue and lethargy, would also slowly dissipate. Side effects from my having fibromyalgia would appear around the six-month mark post-treatment. In short, I was on the bumpy road to recovery.

But there was still the start of tamoxifen to deal with. My medical plan changed again, requiring me to change oncologists. Bummer! The new plan included oncologist Dr. A., who was recommended by my breast surgeon and gynecologist. After discussing my extensive medical history and my current physical and emotional state, she suggested I have my liver problem diagnosed before beginning the tamoxifen, and she recommended a return visit in six months.

After that visit, and given all that had happened in the previous seven months, I began to look at the reality of my health, or lack of it. One thing seemed certain: I could not jump back into the stressful life I had come to know. My cancer experience was a profound lesson in what had to change. My "get up and go" had gotten up and left. In Neale Donald Walsch's book *Conversations with God*, he writes, "If I don't go within, I go without." I needed to explore this.

During a visit with my internist, Dr. T., I shared how I was feeling. Her solution was an antidepressant, but it was not a drug I wanted to take. I was angry about the lack of control I had over my body despite a healthy lifestyle and wanting to just live a normal and productive life. Each medical issue had brought about an unwanted "pause" in my life, and I was tired of the constant pauses. My health had become a full-time job, and my calendar was filled with doctor appointments, lab work, and diagnostic procedures. Dr. T. was sympathetic, but did not have any answers for me, except an antidepressant. I left feeling no better than when I came in.

Chronic illness encompasses more than diagnosis and treatment. A lot of time is consumed driving to and from doctors, and between traffic problems, parking-space hassles, and the cost of parking, it becomes a constant drain on your energy and wallet. There are long waits in crowded waiting rooms, then again in examining rooms. Frustration occurs when calling for test and lab results; often, this requires several calls over the course of days because no one calls you back. Rarely, anymore, do you speak directly to a doctor with questions or concerns unless you are insistent. Messages are often not relayed accurately to the doctor, no matter how articulate you are. And then, there are the insurance claims and payments that require time, energy, patience, and perseverance to resolve. And all the while, you're feeling lousy from chronic pain and illness. Overwhelming!

One particularly frustrating day, I read the Northside Hospital brochure, which outlined monthly health events. The word *wellness* caught my eye as I read about The Wellness Community. "The program, provided free of charge, offers support groups, facilitated by licensed psychotherapists, and a variety of education workshops, networking groups, and stress reduction classes to help participants learn that they are not alone in their fight for recovery." I called and spoke to the program director, Carolyn Helmer, who is now also the executive director. She listened as I poured my heart out, confiding that, for the first time in my life, I felt like isolating myself to avoid the constant explanations of my health. I told her how different I felt from other people. I was blessed with the "looks" of good health—I have always taken a great deal of pride in my appearance.

I wondered if joining a support group would help. I felt led to The Wellness Community, although I knew there were other support groups available to me for other chronic conditions I had. When I finally gave Carolyn a chance to speak, she kindly and gently threw me the "lifeline" I was looking for. She invited me to come to the breast-cancer support group meeting that week. I thanked her for listening to me, and hung up the phone, feeling a sense of peace. I hadn't felt this good in a long while. Two days later, I attended my first support group meeting at The Wellness Community. I immediately liked the group's facilitator, Dede Malpass, with her friendly and gentle manner. In telling us about the history of The Wellness Community, she mentioned that the late comedienne/actress Gilda Radner had participated in the very first one in California. I had a serendipitous moment. Since 1989, when Gilda Radner's book, *It's Always Something,* was published, my life, even up to that point, reflected the title. I still look at her picture on the cover and try to mimic her saying, "Ya know, Jane, it's always something"—a constant reminder of the importance of humor in the midst of adversity.

I immediately felt a bond with the support group as we shared our stories, talking the same language and finding commonality in our breast-cancer experiences, despite the diversity of the group. We came from different parts of the country and were from varying economic backgrounds, races, and religions, but we were all looking for support and answers.

As I told my story, I admitted that I was in a deep well of despair and felt a great deal of anger, guilt, and depression. To avoid constant explanation to family and friends, I isolated myself more and more. My old gregarious self was withdrawing—I was less social than ever. My "normal" life had become increasingly difficult to maintain. I noticed several understanding nods. Realizing that I was not alone,

I felt comforted knowing these women were also struggling with how to go on with their lives. Somewhere I had read that *imbalance creates conflict, which can cause disease.* I needed to change my life.

We all discussed our various treatments—several women were on tamoxifen—and we agreed there was a place for both Western and Eastern medicine in our survival plan. I told of my acupuncture treatments and the practitioner of Chinese medicine I was seeing. When the two-hour meeting was over, Dede had us stand in a circle, holding hands to pause . . . to just . . . breathe. Slowly inhaling and exhaling, I knew I would come back. Through laughter and tears, we had reached out to one another in friendship and sisterhood. What a blessing to have this kind of support in my life. Perhaps now the veil of despair would be lifted.

Eight months post-radiation therapy, I was still tired and lethargic, and still did not have a concrete diagnosis of my liver problem—my doctors had differing opinions. As a result, I had not begun taking tamoxifen. The radiation-treated breast was still pink, swollen, and sore, as was the area under my arm. Pain occurred in my right forearm and hand, extending to my last two fingers, with numbness and tingling. Being right-handed, it was painful to even hold a glass of water. I saw my surgeon, who referred me for evaluation to Robbie Burney, a physical therapist whose specialty is lymphedema. Believe it or not, initially my internist had diagnosed the pain as tennis elbow, knowing I played *no* sports!

Although a mild case, I learned I had lymphedema, and although the daily diuretic I was taking for other medical reasons helped prevent excessive fluid retention, it did not prevent the pain. Diuretics actually exacerbate lymphedema by causing an increased concentration of the stagnant proteins in the tissue, which bind water. Robbie said that she could keep it from progressing any further and gave me three different bandages (similar to an ace bandage) and demonstrated how to wrap my arm. She recommended wearing the bandages as much as possible to decrease the fluid in my lymphatic system and stop the pain. Unfortunately, my sensitive skin reacted just as it had to the tapes on my breast. Intense itching would wake me in the middle of the night, and I'd undo the bandages as fast as I could to scratch my arm. Robbie tried placing a cotton sleeve over my arm first, then putting a piece of foam in the crease of my elbow before wrapping the bandages. Nothing worked until I began applying cortisone cream— the same cream I had used to ease the effects of radiation on my breast—in the crease of my arm before wrapping it.

I was also given exercises to do at home to help keep the fluid from building up and allow for more range of motion. However, the manual massage of my lymphatic system only increased pain in my chest and shoulder area, which led Robbie to suggest another visit to Dr. S. to make sure nothing new had occurred. *Another* diagnosis. This time it was a familiar arthritic condition I had been diagnosed with years before (along with fibromyalgia) called Costochondritis. It causes inflammation in the cartilage where the ribs and breastbone connect. Robbie thought it best to stop the massages. But I continued wrapping my arm and doing my home exercises. One day I will be pain-free. One day.

*   *   *   *   *

Two years have passed since I was treated for breast cancer. My breast healed and lightened in color, and the scar from the lumpectomy is hardly noticeable. I still struggle with pain in my right arm, chest, and shoulder, but am learning to "live with it," along with my other conditions. After a long, arduous road, my liver ailment was diagnosed as a "plumbing" problem within the ducts of the liver. I underwent a liver biopsy followed by enlargement of the common bile duct for a second time in three years. A temporary stent was placed in the duct to hopefully keep it open and unobstructed. Eight weeks later the stent was removed. Although I still experience periodic pain with elevated liver enzymes, it does not occur as often as it did.

At my oncologist's urging, I finally agreed to try taking tamoxifen. I pray for its benefits without any harmful side effects.

To our delight, David and I are now the grandparents of three new babies—in three years! We are doubly blessed that our children live nearby and we can watch those beloved grandchildren grow up.

I made a very difficult decision not to return to work, but remain "in life" as much as possible, enjoying my family and friends.

The Wellness Community continues to provide me with the lifeline for continued hope and perseverance in my survival. The support, love, and special friendships I have made have enriched my life more than words can say. They helped me through some difficult, life-altering decisions, and I've been inspired by the many courageous women I have met. Sadly, several have lost their fight to this dreadful disease, but I am honored to have known them and cherish the special memories I have of each of them.

I am honored to have been invited to speak on behalf of The Wellness Community. It is a pleasure to tell people about this oasis of hope—it has certainly been that for me.

Along with remarkable individuals at The Wellness Community who have meant so much to me, there are numerous classes that enlighten and uplift. Exploring Dreamwork is fascinating and has taught me to "see" a whole new world. I worked through my anger on paper in Recovery Through Art, relieved to know I needed no innate artistic talent! T'ai Chi and yoga classes showed me how to breathe properly and become more focused on a quieter inner self, which helps me cope during stressful days. I learned visualization techniques to relax my mind and body, and fed my spirit by attending Spirituality and Cancer classes. My favorite "fun" event at The Wellness Community is the Joke Fest, where we are encouraged to bring a joke to share—we laugh throughout the evening. It's a well-known and proven fact that laughter produces healthy endorphins which, in turn, boost the body's immune system. Joke Fest judges award prizes for different joke categories, and I have often been a winner. How's this for comic relief:

> A married couple of fifty years are sitting at the breakfast table and the husband says to his wife, "Just think, honey, we've been married for fifty years."
>
> "Yeah," she replies, "fifty years ago we were sitting here at this breakfast table together."
>
> The husband says, "We were probably sitting here naked as jaybirds fifty years ago."
>
> The wife snickers, "What do you say . . . should we get naked?" Whereupon the two strip to the buff, and again sit down at the table. Breathlessly the wife says, "Honey, my nipples are as hot for you today as they were fifty years ago."
>
> "I wouldn't be surprised," replies her husband. "One's in your coffee and the other is in your oatmeal!"

This joke was a grand prize winner.

*   *   *   *   *

Through a lifetime of survivorship, the following comforts me daily in the continuum of life:

Good morning, this is God
I will be handling all your problems today
I will not need your help . . . so, have a good day.

Robin is unable to work, due to her long-standing health problems. She had hoped to complete her five years on tamoxifen, but adverse side effects forced her to discontinue its use after eight months. At present, Robin is cancer-free.

Marion Horton

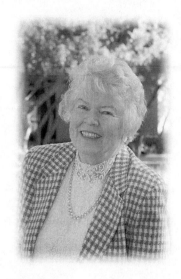

*was born and raised in Savannah,
Georgia. She has been happily married
to her high school sweetheart for fifty-
five years. While raising her four children, she worked as an executive
manager with Tupperware® for twenty-
five years and was often asked to speak
at national conventions, before retiring
in 1991. She and her husband make
frequent trips to their getaway home in
Panama City, Florida. She enjoys family
get-togethers with her children, nine
grandchildren, and most recent addition
to the family, her first great-grandchild.
Marion looks forward each spring to gardening at her suburban
Atlanta home. She is active in her church, where she teaches a
women's Bible study class.*

DIAGNOSIS PROFILE

Age at diagnosis:	55 years old
Family history:	None
Symptoms:	None—abnormal mammogram
Surgery:	Partial radical mastectomy
Biopsy results:	Multifocal infiltrating ductal carcinoma
	Nodes: 19 negative
Therapy:	No further treatment
Second occurrence:	
Age at diagnosis:	72 years old
Symptoms:	None—abnormal mammogram
Surgery:	Needle biopsy
	Lumpectomy
Biopsy results:	Ductal carcinoma in situ (DCIS)
	Stage: 0
	Tumor size: 1.3 cm.
	Nodes: none removed
	Grade: 1
Therapy:	No further treatment
Additional cancer:	
Age at diagnosis:	73 years old
Symptoms:	Vaginal bleeding
Surgery:	D&C
	Total hysterectomy
Biopsy results:	Endometrial cancer
Treatment:	No further treatment

*Anxiety does not empty tomorrow of its sorrows,
it empties today of its strength.*

—Charles Spurgeon

Maybe It Will Go Away

MARION HORTON

A continuing story . . .

In 1984, I went for my routine yearly mammogram and received the usual instructions to call back in a week for the results. Mine was a typical beginning to a continuing breast-cancer story. There is no such thing as a "routine" yearly mammogram.

My mother-in-law, Elizabeth, had died earlier that year as a direct result of chemotherapy. She had stopped smoking about twenty years earlier when she underwent heart bypass surgery, so when a small spot appeared on her lung, we were surprised. Although it was malignant, the doctor did not recommend surgery, but suggested a round of chemo to prevent its spread. He assured us she would die of natural causes long before this tumor got big enough to be threatening. She did well on chemotherapy for two weeks, then had a setback that required hospitalization. She came home still not doing well, but the doctor said her problems were routine, and he would slow down the chemo. When Elizabeth had to go back to the hospital that weekend, she never came home again. They put her on a ventilator but it did not help; she died within a few days. The doctor then said that some people cannot handle the chemo and the way it impacts their system. Evidently she was one of those people. He seemed quite unconcerned but, in effect, said that the chemo was the cause of her death.

That was a terrible time for us. My husband, Claude, and I had believed the doctor and expected his mother to have many more years. She was in good health and enjoyed, among other things, driving to Atlanta to see our family. We were all raised in Savannah, and Elizabeth was never able to accept the fact that we had left, especially to move to the "far country."

On one of our trips to Savannah to see my mother-in-law, our daughter withheld information about her own physical condition. Melanie had recently had a miscarriage, but chose not to tell us. She thought we had enough to worry about. The doctor discovered she had a hydatidiform mole requiring a D&C. This is a highly aggressive form of a precancerous condition. Melanie's doctor told her it could spread to her liver, her lungs, and anywhere else. If a D&C did not remove it completely, she'd need another one in a month. He did not say what would happen after that. Melanie and her husband, Bill, were quite devastated. They had three young children, and Melanie was even thinking of instructions to leave for her husband's next wife if this mole turned into the unthinkable. She assumed he could not raise three children without help, so another wife would likely be a necessity. Both Melanie and Bill went to the Lord in prayer. Bill belonged to a men's group who prayed many hours for Melanie's healing. My daughter and son-in-law both received a peace about it, knowing she was in the hands of someone much more capable than mere mortal doctors. When she went back to the doctor a month after her D&C, he could not find anything in her blood indicating she had even had this condition! She was required to return at six-month intervals for the next two years, but she had no further signs of anything wrong. Praise God!

My father-in-law's death from colon cancer was preceded by my husband's brother's brief bout with pancreatic cancer. His demise, at the age of forty-eight, meant the loss of three members of Claude's immediate family in less than a year—his mother, father, and brother. It was a tough time for both of us. And with all this tragedy to deal with, I certainly was not concerned about the results of a mammogram that had been normal for many years. Each time we left the city limits, I would remember that I hadn't phoned the doctor's office about my mammogram results, but when I was home, the thought never entered my mind. After several weeks, it became embarrassing to think of calling, and besides, if anything was wrong, they would have called me, right? Wrong!

My son Craig, a pediatrician, was in the Air Force and had recently been transferred to the Philippines. He and his wife, Debbie, were expecting their first child. One evening, he called to say they had a little boy, born that morning with great difficulty, but everything turned out well. Then, a very surprising admission came from my son the pediatrician and his wife, a pediatric nurse. He said in a hushed tone, almost a whisper, "Mama, we don't know what to do with this baby!" He and Debbie were overwhelmed. He was so emotional. Of course, now that they lived so far away, no family was with them. Even Debbie's mother, who did not like to fly, had not planned to go.

The next morning, Sunday, I said to my husband, "You know what?"

He said, "Yes, I know what."

I said, "You do not."

He said, "You want to go to the Philippines."

Claude was right, of course. We went to church, still in turmoil, and mentioned it to my Bible study class. Someone told us where we could quickly get a passport. Guess who was there early that same afternoon? Before dark, all my papers were filled out, picture taken, everything I needed. Now it had to be hand-carried to somewhere in Washington, D.C. to be completed. I was assured it would be back by Monday afternoon. The cost of a passport through normal channels was around $20, but it usually took about two months. This one cost $225, but was less than two days in the making. By Monday morning, my husband and my son had decided it was not safe for me to travel alone, so Claude began the passport process immediately. My passport came back that Monday afternoon, his arrived on Tuesday, and we were on a plane to the Philippines on Wednesday morning.

Landing at the airport in Manila was unlike anything we had ever experienced—a complete culture shock. There appeared to be thousands of people, all shoving and pushing, no carousels from which to retrieve luggage, only a chute. This "thing" dumped everything all over the floor of the airport and a mad scramble ensued. They were right, I would not have made it alone! Craig wasn't even allowed to come into the terminal to help us with the luggage. Have I mentioned that there were no skycaps either? We finally were able to find our things, all mashed and buried in all the other luggage. It was difficult to carry everything, but we made it out of the airport and to the curb where Craig was parked. I was surprised to see Debbie in the front seat—after all, she had just given birth four days earlier. They had traveled all the way from Clark Air Base, over narrow, bumpy roads, for an hour and a half. Nothing prepared me for the next surprise, one of the best of my entire life. When I opened the back door of the car, there on the seat, lying very quietly, wrapped in a blanket, was Alex, our newest grandson! His mother did not want us to have to wait to see him. I cried. Claude and I were both overjoyed.

Since Claude was in business for himself as a concrete contractor and I was a Tupperware manager, we were fortunate to be able to take three weeks off to be with them. Of course, when you are your own boss, your income stops when you leave town. Craig had offered to pay our plane fare, but since Claude refused to let him, Craig paid all our expenses while we were there, including buying all the souvenirs we brought back. Prices were so unbelievably low we were able to bring home many beautiful things. Sightseeing was an exciting part of our visit, and we were lucky enough to see numerous places that are no longer there since the volcanic eruption in 1989 that almost wiped out the entire base. Sadly, before the United States could rebuild the air base, the Philippine government decided they no longer wanted our people there, and so, in addition to the air base leaving, it was not long before the naval base was gone too.

Debbie was concerned when Claude and I volunteered to get up during the night and take care of Alex. She whispered to Craig, wondering if the baby's bottle would be warm enough and if we would remember to change him. I think she probably stayed awake all night worrying. *Worry* is definitely the right word. Alex is now seventeen, and she still worries about him, even though the young man is never sick. Then again, when your dad is a doctor, it doesn't really matter, does it?

Our visit with Craig and Debbie took place in August, which meant I had to cancel my reservations for the annual Tupperware convention, a first for me. I never missed those gatherings of thousands of people from all over America—they were too much fun. Also, the women who are in sales are recognized with many wonderful incentives. I always made it my business to be included among those who were well rewarded with leather luggage, trips, cruises, fur coats, etc. In my twenty-five years with Tupperware, most of them as an executive manager, I qualified for many of these awards. In fact, we had a trip to Acapulco coming up in September.

Now back to my unknown test results. I had simply forgotten about it. I had so many other things on my mind. And I was really not concerned about a test that I was certain would be normal. Ironically, in recent months I had discovered a sign in one of my doctor's reception areas that read: "MIWGA: Maybe It Will Go Away." The sign pointed out that these five words are the most dangerous to a woman's health. Just as I shrugged off the possibility that something could be terribly wrong with me, other women did the same. Tragically, this nonchalant attitude of denial has led to many deaths.

My doctor called me in September. It seems he was making plans to retire in November and was cleaning off his desk and noticed we had not spoken regarding my test results. He said my mammogram showed some abnormalities and that I should come in immediately. When I did, he showed me the film. There were three tiny pinpoint spots—the size of the *point* of a pin, not the head. He said that when they begin to get "friendly" and clump together, there could be trouble. They were so tiny, however, he said it would likely be five or six years before they would be big enough to be felt, so we were getting it early. *It?* You mean "it" already has a name?

On the following Monday, when I reported to the hospital for a biopsy, I was quite annoyed at this whole inconvenience. As the nurse prepared me for the needle localization, she commented offhandedly, "Eighty percent of these things are benign. I don't think you have anything to worry about." *What?* You mean I have a 20 percent chance for a malignancy! That's when I began to get a little worried. The three wires she placed in my breast were quite painful. She said she could anesthetize the surface, but could not get it far enough inside to completely deaden the pain of the wire insertion. At the time, my breasts were quite dense, so this was not a fun procedure. Understatement. The ends of the wires sort of waved around while I was being wheeled to the operating room. This was a lot to go through, but I did want the doctor to know exactly where these three infinitesimal spots were. Wouldn't want to have to repeat this.

Late in the afternoon, I was awakened by the doctor asking me, "Are you awake?" Still half asleep, I was annoyed by the necessity of this procedure so I answered, "No." This was a silly attitude, wasn't it? It wasn't the doctor's fault that this thing had grown in me, but at this moment he was the bad guy. He returned about an hour later and bluntly announced, "There is a malignancy. I have scheduled you for a mastectomy on Thursday." With that, he left.

When I broke the news to my sister, Dolores, in Jacksonville, she was visibly upset, telling me this was not a "plain vanilla" situation and that I needed to take it seriously. She and her husband are part of a broad prayer network, and they put me at the top of their list. I needed it. Dolores is my only sister, and we have always been very close. There is less than two years difference in our ages. We used to double-date; we were married exactly a year apart; we'd had our children at the same time. Our first two boys were eighteen days apart, the second two boys nine days apart. Our mother said if we had two more boys, she was going to head into the woods. We then had baby girls just twenty-one days apart, but her infant girl died at birth, when mine was three weeks old. This tragic event was followed by a blessing, when Dolores had a perfect baby girl just sixteen months later. So each of our children had a cousin of a similar age. Of course, when my "extra dividend" came along thirteen years later, Dolores said to me, "Kid, I'm not going to join you this time. You're on your own."

My cancer diagnosis was taken in stride by my mother who admonished me not to be so concerned. My brother, Dick, came right over with a hug and a promise to see that I got anything and everything necessary to make this thing go away. Dolores remained extremely upset.

Claude and I had planned to leave in a week for Acapulco, a much-anticipated trip earned through Tupperware Home Parties. I called the doctor's office to ask if we could delay the surgery a week, hoping we would be able to travel a week early to Acapulco. With my doctor's consent, my wonderful friend and distributor, Ray, made arrangements through our home office in Florida. Claude and I were on our way to Mexico the very next morning. Because the plans were changed at the last minute, the girl in our Orlando office called me back to ask, "Now why did I make these changes for you?" I explained what I was facing when I returned. She was so sweet and sympathetic, saying she would alert the tour guides so that anything I needed would be provided. She also said she'd ask the entire office to include me in their prayers. At that time, she did not know me at all, but a very personal friendship developed over the course of the next few months. She called me after my surgery and said she would pass on the good news that it had gone well to the rest of the office. I shall always remember her kindness.

On our second day in Acapulco, my biopsied breast began to swell and turned a very dark purple—almost black, and ached accordingly. The only way to reach my doctor was to place a collect call to his home, which I did. Though he was not a personal friend, just my surgeon, his wife was in my Bible study class. She answered the phone, immediately accepting the charges. When he came on the line, he said the swelling was a result of the biopsy and that I needed to see a doctor. He reconsidered when I reminded him where I was. He recommended hot, wet towels and to hope for the best. Eventually the swelling began to subside and the pain lessened. I didn't worry much about it. After all, they were cutting it off the next week anyway!

As if this wasn't enough excitement for one week, suddenly a hurricane appeared. We were marooned at our hotel, The Acapulco Princess. The lower floor flooded, but it was on ground level. There were no walls; you just walked in through a beautiful garden that continued all through the lobby. There was lots of mopping up, but apparently no danger. The hotel set up game rooms, and furnished impromptu entertainment for the guests. Tupperware had an entire room for the fifteen couples that had qualified for this "trip of a life-time." We played games, ate snacks, and just talked and enjoyed our-selves. One of the other ladies there told me that if I did require chemotherapy, frozen grapes would help relieve the nausea. Someone else gave me the address of a good place to buy wigs that was near Atlanta. They were all so attentive. The hurricane over, we were soon sightseeing, shopping, enjoying the beach, and watching cliff divers for the rest of the week. I had only one regret: I was not in any condition to enjoy the parasails. On a previous trip to Acapulco, I had loved the feeling of freedom as I sailed high above the rooftops and over the beautiful beach. When it was time to leave and everyone was saying their goodbyes, many couples promised to remember me in their prayers. I was very grateful because I know that prayer makes you stronger.

When you are facing surgery, any previous operations you've had come to mind. When surgery was required to realign the bones in my feet, the doctor would only do them one at a time, about two to three weeks apart. My feet had caused me pain all my life, so this was to be a wonderful outcome. I scheduled the second surgery to be completed before our yearly Tupperware Spring Sessions. Since I was in sales, it was a challenge to be recognized in the top group among others across the country. I had always made it my business to be there, and this time would be no exception. I was excited. The top people were rewarded handsomely, not only in dollars, but with incentives like our trip to Acapulco, along with tangible gifts such as refrigerators, washers, and fine china, to name a few. My entire house was furnished by Tupperware!

But this Tupperware convention was not to be. Two weeks after the surgery, when the second foot should have been operated on, I was back in the hospital with an infection that had dug a hole in the top of my foot all the way to the bone. Each day the doctor would come in, poke around in the hole, declaring its apparent inability to heal itself. After ten days, the doctor sent me home, but since I was on crutches and unable to travel, I missed the convention.

On another occasion, I had scheduled surgery well before an important event—we were about to celebrate our fiftieth wedding anniversary. This time it was a cataract, simple, easily removed and recovered from. The eye that needed the surgery had endured a vitrectomy three years earlier. This procedure removes the vitreous fluid from behind the eye and replaces it with a saline solution. The surgeon asked if I wanted to be put to sleep, and when he explained what he would be doing, I answered, "No."

I foolishly thought I'd be able to watch what he was doing. The first thing they did was cover my entire face with a dark surgical drape. As I listened while he worked, he kept exclaiming, "This thing is really hard. It doesn't want to break up." He was using more force than I had anticipated, but there was no pain, just pressure. As he continued to make comments, I asked if the fact I'd had a vitrectomy made any difference. He said, "Of course, I forgot that!" Whoa, he *forgot* that? I think I'm in trouble.

I suddenly recalled reading about a different procedure in some of the literature he had given me during a previous visit to his office. I asked him about it. He said no, that we were okay. *Uh-oh.* He then said, "Deep six. I was afraid of that." Those were his exact words. I will never forget them. I knew what he had done. He had pushed the cataract into the back of my eye. We were now over an hour and a half into a procedure that should have taken less than a half hour.

As a result of that "unfortunate outcome," I have only a small amount of peripheral vision in my right eye. The middle of my line of sight is black, no way to ever fix it. Of course, after this debacle, the eye required another vitrectomy in order to remove the cataract.

This surgery was such a strange recovery. It was just my eye, but every bone in my body was affected. There was a great deal of shooting pain and burning, with no improvement in my vision. I kept a diary of this event—daily feelings, doctor visits, results, or rather, lack of results.

A week after the cataract surgery, the doctor said the tear ducts were clogged, causing the pressure to rise in my eye. He could open them up with his laser. It would only take a few minutes. It was the most horrendous few minutes I have ever spent—sort of what I would imagine surgery without anesthesia would feel like. He put a block of wood in my eye to hold it open, then shot the laser. It felt like a bullet. I screamed. He said, "Only a little bit more." He hit it several more times with the laser: it was pure torture. Then he asked the nurse a question to which she answered, "I thought *you* did." It seems each one thought the other had anesthetized my eye, and neither had! Even after the deadening agent was administered, it was still awful. The laser would not go through. The doctor finally became annoyed with the machine and shot it like a machine gun into my eye. Some of his comments were similar to the ones during the operation. "I can't understand this." "What is the problem?" "Something is wrong." There definitely was something wrong!

When the doctor checked the pressure in my eye, it was much too high and we could not schedule the vitrectomy to remove the cataract from behind the eye until the pressure came down, swelling diminished, and I felt I could tolerate the additional surgery. That turned out to be two more weeks of pure misery. On the day before the vitrectomy was scheduled, the eye was bright red, burning like a wildfire, and I was so sick that the ophthalmologist said, "We can't wait any longer." I only spent one night in the hospital and came home with my eye patched, which is the way it stayed until the day before our anniversary reception.

On our big day, I was barely able to stand alone. Only by the grace of God was my eye open. Despite all this, our reception was absolutely glorious, so many people—all of our children and all but two of the grandchildren were there—an event to remember forever. One of my dear Tupperware friends had written our entire fifty years in verse. Our oldest son, Steve, then read what he had written, which was, as always, hilarious. Steve is the one, who, when he was a freshman at Georgia Tech, came home for the first time from college to discover a new trash compactor and commented, "It didn't take you long to replace me." For the reception, our daughter, Melanie, sang "Always," which had been sung at our wedding. She has her father's beautiful, high, clear voice. I felt so blessed to see so many beloved people together for such a happy occasion. Everyone knew the trauma I had just experienced and assured me I looked fine. I knew better.

* * * *

When we got the news from my doctor that there was a malignancy in my breast, our son Craig received emergency leave through the Red Cross and arrived from the Philippines by the time I was scheduled for surgery. Debbie and baby Alex came, too. Debbie's mother was finally able to see her first grandchild. We returned from Acapulco on a Tuesday, and I went into the hospital that night. On Wednesday morning, Craig came in to see the doctor with his father and me. The doctor said a spot this size would take five to six years to get large enough to be felt. We discussed lumpectomy instead of the partial radical mastectomy he prescribed. The doctor said I was not a candidate for lumpectomy because of the cancer's location and that was that. He did not discuss it further. We thought he assumed I was too old for a lumpectomy to make a difference. I was fifty-five. We did not question his judgment.

Sometimes I wish we had, and sometimes I am glad we did not. With a lumpectomy, there is often radiation and sometimes chemotherapy. And the chance of missing a rogue cell or two. At the time, we didn't know what I was facing.

Craig asked if he could be in the operating room during my surgery. My doctor said he did not think that was a good idea since it would be his mother who was undergoing major surgery. We accepted that.

I was grateful that my children were close by. Our oldest son, Steve, and his family had just relocated to Atlanta from Tucson, Arizona. Our daughter, Melanie, with husband Bill, and their then three children (now four) lived near us. And we still had our youngest son, Matt, a high-schooler, at home. Matt said later that he hardly knew what exactly was going on—that nobody ever told him anything!

After the surgery, my surgeon informed me that he'd left enough tissue and skin so that I could have reconstruction if I decided to do so in the future. The procedure had a novel way of shifting fat from your belly to form your new breast. I certainly had an ample source, but when I investigated what the additional surgery involved, I determined that it was too much of an ordeal for me. I have never looked back.

My incision from the partial radical mastectomy went from just below my breast diagonally through the armpit and two inches down my arm. They removed nineteen lymph nodes, all of which were negative; therefore, no chemo and no radiation needed. Home free, right? I had family and many friends who reminded me how lucky I was for the positive outcome. Everyone was rejoicing that the doctor "got it all," yet I was experiencing feelings of depression. I didn't tell anyone how I really felt, though.

The American Cancer Society sent my friend Martha Knighton to see me with the gift of a temporary prosthesis and literature about it. She told me that she'd had a radical mastectomy some twenty years before when she was in her early thirties. This was news to me.

At that time, when this operation was performed, doctors removed so much chest muscle that she was literally concave on one side. She had me feel her breasts to see if I could tell which side was real and which was the prosthesis. I refused at first, but she insisted. (I have since found myself doing the same thing to others. People are hesitant, of course, but when they do, it is a revelation to them that both sides feel the same.) I still was not convinced. Martha told me many helpful things that I could never have imagined. She talked about my husband and his possible reactions—she even covered the subject of sex. What a surprise! We talked about a mutual friend who had undergone a double mastectomy. Her husband had left her, and the divorce was even more traumatic than the loss of her breasts. Martha also told me of a support group I might be interested in attending. All this was so very new to me, it was hard to take everything in. Martha came to see me again the next morning. She must have known how important that second visit was. She was an enormous help, as I know she must have been to many others, since she not only represented the American Cancer Society, but could also speak from personal experience.

Yellow roses are so expensive. They were then and they are now, but nevertheless, they are my favorite. They've come with all the babies, other operations, special occasions, and sometimes "just because." This time, Claude bought me diamonds instead. They were a bit more costly than yellow roses, but I have enjoyed wearing those earrings since the ordeal seventeen years ago. Yellow roses don't last that long.

My second night in the hospital, I was sick of hearing how lucky I was. By then the pain had settled in to the point that it seemed to think it belonged there and would just remain forever. Pain medication was not much help. All my visitors had left, it was a few minutes after 11:00 p.m. When the new night nurse, Carol Cohen, arrived to check on me, she found me crying. Everyone knows how busy these nurses are, especially during shift changes, so I certainly did not expect her to be concerned. But she was. Carol came in, sat on the bed, and asked how she could help. When she found out how guilty I felt about feeling sorry for myself, she was quick to point out that I had every reason to feel that way. After all, I had undergone major surgery, which is never a picnic. My body was scarred forever, which, she said, required some mourning. A part of my body was missing. I had certainly never thought of it that way. Carol said I would live with this loss every day for the rest of my life. She asked about my husband. Some husbands are in such a state of shock themselves that they don't get over this traumatic change. I assured her that I had the best husband, and he loved me devotedly, happy with whatever was left of me. Carol asked if I had eaten dinner, and when I told her I hadn't been hungry, she was able to find some chicken soup and crackers, which helped a lot. She continued to stay and talk to me, and I truly believe she saved my sanity. I have never been able to properly thank her. Until now.

Compassion in the medical field means so much. On two occasions, when I accompanied Craig on his hospital rounds, I observed how he did circumcisions. He placed what appeared to be a heavy metal circle on the baby's penis, then turned around to talk to me. After a few minutes, he finished the procedure. The nurse told me that Dr. Horton, my son, was the only doctor she had ever known who allowed the cold of the metal to take effect and lessen the pain that the baby felt. It takes a little longer, but certainly is worth it. We went into the room of a nine-month-old who had been admitted for breathing problems. Craig picked her up from the crib, talked with her mother, then turned to the baby and said, "Now, Emily, I want you to know that when a nurse comes in with a needle, Dr. Horton had nothing to do with it." He handed the baby to her mother and left quickly as the nurse entered the room.

On return visits to my doctor, before I was fitted for a prosthesis, we laughed at my falling over sideways when I walked. When you have a crooked body, that's the way you walk. My recovery was faster than I had expected, within four weeks I was as back to normal as anyone would have thought possible. I was driving all over the city and picking up my Tupperware parties right where I had left off.

I went for my first prosthesis fitting about four weeks after surgery. Nancy Wells of The Tender Touch was recommended to me, and she is still my favorite fitter. When Nancy had a mastectomy in 1978, she was disappointed in the lack of qualified people available to fit prostheses. She also missed the availability of a shop that carried clothing and accessories for mastectomy patients, so she opened her own. I love the name The Tender Touch—so apropos. The shop sells bathing suits and nightgowns with breast pockets in them to hold the form securely. She first fitted the bra, then found the breast form that most closely matched my missing one. The bra's soft pockets on both sides comfortably accommodate both the real side and the "fake" side. When Nancy put a tight, knitted, striped shirt on me, I laughed. She immediately assured me that I would not likely be wearing this in public, but it showed the correct fit. If the stripes were crooked, adjustments were necessary. She fixed it all, making me feel very comfortable, thanks to her talent and her attitude. To quote Nancy, "Attitude is everything!"

Prostheses are funny things: They are heavy, but then again they are supposed to replace a part of your body that was heavy, depending on your breast size. They are not at all uncomfortable; they're soft, sort of wiggly, and not at all like anything you have ever seen or felt before.

This may sound strange, but there are times when a prosthesis comes in rather handy. I assume that any female with extra weight on board would do just about anything to show fewer pounds on her medical chart. At the doctor's office, the nurse always wants to know my weight. As I dutifully step onto the scale, I often will reach under my blouse, remove my prosthesis, and hand my portable breast to the nurse. She usually laughs and deducts two pounds.

Prostheses have improved over the years. For one thing, even though they still have weight, they are lighter and more comfortable. Several years ago, I was excited to obtain a new form that sticks to the body with the help of skin supports. The support stays on the skin for about a week before it is necessary to apply a new one. I expected this to be helpful when in a swimming pool, but I discovered that I still needed a bra. However, Nancy supplied me with swim forms, which were great. Before she advised me of the availability of swim forms, Claude and I were swimming in a motel pool in Florida when we spotted my prosthesis floating halfway down the pool! It looked like a jellyfish that had lost its way. Luckily, it was late in the evening and we were the only ones in the water. He rescued it while I nearly drowned with laughter. The prostheses that are now available do not require skin supports, but simply stick to the skin with little suction cups. Some women who are very small breasted and don't really need a bra, have welcomed this improvement.

My group insurance policy that covered Tupperware managers turned out to be excellent coverage. We were very pleased. Our pleasure didn't last long, however. When Tupperware switched insurance carriers, the new carrier excluded me from the group policy. All of a sudden, Claude and I had no medical coverage. (Claude was included on my policy since he was self-employed.) Now nobody would take me no matter what the price. It was almost three years before we finally found an insurance company that would take a chance on me. And there were so many exclusions in this coverage, it was hardly worth the exorbitant cost.

A few months after my surgery, I discovered two very large, hard lumps under my arm. Panic! Early one morning, I called my doctor, saying that I would meet him on any street corner immediately.

Later that morning, at his office, he checked the lumps and reassured me they were just part of my arm and had been there all along. Whew! I think I was more frightened this time than at any other—I thought the cancer had come back already, that my life was over. This was at the time when many people were going to the Bahamas for laetrile treatment for all kinds of cancers, some claiming to be cured. Claude and I were considering doing this while driving to the doctor's office, along with anything else anyone might suggest. It's ironic how, when you face your mortality, you'll try anything.

Back then, there were not many support groups, but I didn't feel that I needed one; my husband loved me. He had said to the doctor that he would take any piece of me that was left, just fix whatever was wrong. Claude has always been this way. My mother picked him out for me in third grade. He was the smartest boy in the class and always wore a white shirt and tie to school. This was in the late 1930s—things were very different then. He moved after that school year, but we met up again in junior high school, where we ran against each other for seventh-grade vice-president. He won! In ninth grade, we ran against each other again. This time, I won. And this time, it was for president of the student council, which automatically made him vice-president. We worked quite closely together, and the following year we were required to help with the installation of the new officers. It was about the time of the annual Harvest Ball. Claude's sister insisted he take me. We both dated others for a short while, but by the time we were sixteen, it was a permanent arrangement. The rest is history. My four children and nine grandchildren are a very precious part of my life, but my husband *is* my life.

In 1984, breast-cancer support groups were few and far between. I did find one, and it was surprisingly helpful. I learned that others were having the same problems I was: tightness under the arm, feeling uncomfortable in clothing, etc. The tightness lasted approximately five years. Each time I mentioned it to my doctor, his response (since this was not life-threatening) was always the same: "It'll go away." It did, eventually.

Over the next few years, two additional biopsies were required, both benign. No more problems.

*   *   *   *   *

When my mother was ninety, she asked me to look at a very hard lump just below her shoulder. She lived alone, and her bedroom was on the second floor of her condo, requiring her to climb stairs several times a day. She enjoyed cooking occasionally for my brother and his wife, and sometimes baby-sat the great-grandchildren. In other words, she was very independent. She told me she had slipped going upstairs one day and had hit her shoulder on the banister. The lump I felt was quite alarming, about the size of a peach pit. Never once did it occur to me that cancer sometimes shows up that way. I took her to her doctor, who sent us to a breast specialist. A breast specialist! What on earth for?

It was my opportunity to meet one of the most caring doctors I have ever known. I did not know at the time that *I'd* have use for her services in a few years. She was so kind to my mother, listened to her as she felt the lump, and agreed it must have been a hard fall. She insisted on doing a mammogram, my mother's first. This was followed by a needle aspiration, which told us nothing. When I questioned the necessity of all this, she said breast cancer will oftentimes manifest itself in this manner. Breast cancer! How could that be? The lump was almost on her shoulder and her breasts were almost down around her waist! The doctor convinced me that anything in this area of the chest involves breast tissue. None of this worried my mother at all; she continued to believe the hard lump on her shoulder was the result of her fall. Basically, my mother did not believe the doctor. However, she was convinced when she ended up in the hospital for surgery the following week. The report came back that the lump was malignant, but the doctor said she "got it all," and prescribed tamoxifen. This drug is supposed to suppress a recurrence, right? And my mother is a ninety-year-old now . . . oh, well. She had promised me she'd live to be one hundred, so we went for it. She came through the surgery beautifully, with minimal pain. But she wasn't able to keep her promise. She died at age ninety-four—of a brain tumor.

* * * * *

While enjoying a summer weekend with a group of Tupperware friends, I was struck by an intense pain in the middle of my stomach. It would not stop, and I could not eat. Now, with this group, eating is one of the things we all do best. Each is a better cook than the other, and when we get together, it is a banquet. Thankfully, no one noticed I was not consuming my share. The doctor I went to the next day said it appeared that the umbilical hernia I had had for some time had decided to act up. When this happens, there's a chance of peritonitis as a result of the hernia's becoming strangulated. Surgery would be necessary. For some unknown, ridiculous reason, I thought the incision would be about the size of my navel, since that was where the hernia was, and that this would be a simple operation. Claude had had surgery when he was much younger. I had forgotten his was the kind men get, much lower, and smaller.

When I woke up from this surgery, I had nineteen staples across my middle, and no navel. The doctor said, "I took it out; you didn't need it anyway." Another body part missing. Will this ever end? Oh well, my bikini days were over anyway. But I do wish the surgeon had told me he was going to make my navel disappear before he did it.

* * * * *

Three years later, I felt another lump in the naval area, which sometimes ached. *Oh, no, not again.* When I went back to the surgeon who had repaired the hernia, he verified my suspicions. A friend suggested another surgeon for a second opinion. He recommended a CAT scan to be sure. By then, I was sure. We discussed the use of a permanent mesh to prevent the hernia from breaking loose. He agreed we should use it this time, just so I wouldn't have to go through this again. Hard to believe, but when I woke up and inquired about the mesh, the surgeon said he had not seen the need to use it. There apparently was plenty of room to repair the abdominal wall so that it would not be a problem again. Good. I believed him.

I thought the lump that was still evident in my stomach was too big and brought it up during my follow-up visit. The surgeon's partner, whom I saw this time, assured me it would go away, but it might take six months. It did not "go away." It continued to get bigger. Two months later, it had grown to approximately the size of a baseball, leading me to think that maybe it was something else. By the time it had grown to the size of a softball (seemed like a basketball), it was really beginning to bother me, both the way it felt and the way it looked. A visit to a new doctor confirmed it was the hernia, *again*. He said it was up to me as to when to have another operation. Third doctor, third operation. I was assured by this surgeon that he would not leave out the mesh this time, guaranteed. In my opinion, the second doctor forgot—the same as my eye doctor had done, which resulted in my being blind in one eye.

And if this wasn't enough for one lifetime, my "routine yearly mammogram" had to be looked at again. The test in April came back with the notation "suspicious of malignancy," and the recommendation that I see a surgeon. Remember, I am not a worrier. Things just do not bother me—never have. It never occurs to me that there might be something to worry about. Of course, it does occur to me that if something is seriously wrong, I might not get to see my grandchildren graduate from college, get married, and have families of their own. This unhappy thought lasts just a short time, not something I dwell on. After many years, I have, to a degree, been able to teach this to my husband. Our daughter, an eternal optimist, takes after me. My sons are always very supportive and, as far as I can tell, they always expect the best outcome. And we all, as a family, are very grounded in our faith and always look to Him for support and peace of mind.

On the same day that I met with the doctor regarding my hernia, I saw the breast specialist. This was the one who had been so kind to my mother, and that I never expected to see again. The visit began with a mammogram and ultrasound, even though I brought all the pictures previously taken. The doctor performed a needle biopsy. Though I was not in a position to watch the procedure, Claude described how the screen showed each thrust of the needle, and each little piece of tissue was dropped into a tiny bottle. The test results arrived a week later. A surgical excisional biopsy was now required, meaning a visit to the hospital. This was scheduled for the week prior to the hernia operation, and I wanted to be well enough for it. Since I have a hard time waking up from anesthesia, we asked one of the doctors about the possibility of having both operations at the same time. The answer was, "I don't think so."

Nothing is ever easy. On that day as I was being prepared to go into the operating room and was talking to the surgeon, the anesthesiologist questioned my EKG, which showed a right bundle branch block, as did the one I'd had before the last hernia surgery. He adamantly announced he would not put me to sleep without my first having a stress test and a visit to a cardiologist. So, surgery was cancelled.

The hernia surgery also had to be cancelled, but now both doctors agreed they could operate at the same time! (Now, if only I could find a cooperative knee doctor, we might be able to accomplish a complete overhaul.)

The stress test results confirmed my feeling—they were normal. Then again, my feelings have not been very accurate so far, have they? After some logistical problems in attempting to get two very busy doctors together, we finally settled on a date for the double surgery. I was somewhat concerned, knowing that two months had gone by since this breast problem was discovered.

My breast surgeon had said she would need an hour, the hernia doctor said he would need two hours. Since they were able to work simultaneously, I was only "out" for a total of one hour and forty-five minutes. Great! I was able to go home the next morning.

Needless to say, I had quite a wretched week, but time is a great healer. The following Monday, when I saw both doctors, I received a good report from one and a not-so-good one from the other. Guess which one was "not so good"? Right, the breast report. There were suspicions of something else within the area the doctor removed, and now they were using the words "ductal carcinoma in situ." The lab report was sent out for further study and it would take a week to get the results. Here we go again!

This time I was concerned. When my breast doctor read the report and discovered the possibility of further cancer, she covered her face with the report and said this would probably mean radiation and maybe other treatment, depending on what was found. Up to this point, I had not required anything like this. Claude and I discussed my having to endure the treatment and decided that whatever was necessary, we would face it. My mind was all but made up that radiation was in my immediate future.

On Thursday, Melanie and I had been out having lunch, a weekly mother and daughter event, and we were in a doll shop, "just looking," when her cell phone rang. It was her dad saying he had heard from the doctor. I took the phone and heard him repeat what the doctor said. "She got it all. Call in three months for an appointment." Claude was sobbing! Needless to say, we were all elated. Hallelujah. No radiation! And, of course, the most important thing: *no more cancer.*

When our first three children were little, we had a friend whose three were the same ages as ours. She and her family always went to her in-laws for Sunday dinner each week after church. I did so envy her. I decided right then and there that when mine grew up, I would do the same for them and their families. When Steve was married, he and his wife were invited each week to join us for Sunday dinner after church. That was more than twenty-five years ago, and I still cook for any of the family that is in town. Automatic ovens make it simple, along with preparations made on Saturday. We always go to the eight-thirty church and Bible study, then we're back home by a quarter past eleven to get dinner on the table by one o'clock. Claude helps with everything, including the cleanup afterward. Sometimes we have eight, sometimes twelve, sometimes more, around the dining room table. I wouldn't miss it for the world. It is boisterous and fun and is my chance to interact with the busy people whom I love.

Being "out of commission" from surgery now keeps me from cooking every Sunday, and I miss it more than words can say. Also, this year, due to the timing of my "interruptions," our garden even suffered. We always can lots of tomatoes, snap beans, apples, pears, and fig preserves. This, of course, helps with the grocery bill. Besides, Claude and I love to "dig." Since I could not bend over because of hernia surgery, and couldn't reach up too well either, Claude had to do it all. The weeds got the best of us, alas. But we still harvested lots of good vegetables and fruits, and gave them to friends and neighbors. We did some canning, but not nearly as much as usual, nor nearly as much as we plan to do in the coming year. A cruise with our four children and their spouses is in the works.

Although my experience with The Wellness Community has been minimal, I recently read an article in the *Atlanta Journal-Constitution* that said women live longer when they are a part of a network, a support group. Even the research scientists were stunned to discover that women who attended weekly support group meetings lived twice as long as those who did not. Women are different. They are strong. They are compassionate. You can share your innermost thoughts and fears and find someone who has gone through what you are facing—someone who can help you. The Wellness Community-Atlanta is a good thing.

My next follow-up visit to the breast doctor was uneventful. She said I could return in six months or a year, but since I had "misbehaved twice," she would recommend six months. As always, I expected no more problems.

A year later, as I sat at my sewing machine after a water aerobics class that morning I began having cramps—the kind that usually accompany periods! Then I suddenly discovered that I was bleeding—exactly like a period. I hadn't experienced anything like this in twenty years. The bleeding had not stopped by late afternoon, and since I did not have a gynecologist, Claude drove me to the emergency room of our local hospital. When I told the doctor I was "acting like a teenager," he asked, "Are you sassing your parents, too?" After his examination was over, he recommended I see a gynecologist the next day for further diagnosis. He said I had a possible malignancy. Whoa!

Getting an immediate doctor's appointment is not easy. I called several the next morning—all were heavily booked and couldn't see me right away. I finally got an appointment with my daughter-in-law's gynecologist, who not only saw me that afternoon, he talked to me on the phone—how unusual. How nice. He did a D&C and was almost certain that it was malignant, and that I would require a hysterectomy. Test results would be back in five to seven days. But he called the very next evening, saying he was able to get a faster read and that his suspicions were confirmed. I had endometrial cancer. He offered to pull some strings and was able to get me in to see a gynecological oncologist the very next day.

After all these years, I thought I had dodged the proverbial bullet in not needing a hysterectomy. Unfortunately, I was not a candidate for the less invasive kind, a vaginal hysterectomy. Mine would have to be the abdominal (read: "abominable") kind, which meant more pain, and longer and more difficult recovery. There was, however, an upside to the hysterectomy: while he was at it, the surgeon did a sigmoidoscopy, he took out my appendix and rearranged my intestines, which was necessary because of the previous hernia surgery!

During the five days I spent in the hospital, one knee became so painful I was unable to walk, which was a necessity after any kind of surgery. An orthopedist said it was gout and proceeded to drain the knee. That turned out to be an instant cure, and I was once again upright on both legs.

Recovery was even slower than I had thought it would be. Christmas was only six weeks away and we were expecting our usual big family gathering. Fortunately, I had no trouble allowing my children and grandchildren to pitch in and do everything and, as always, my beloved Claude took great care of me.

Now, let's try again. I am not expecting any more problems and plan to travel, enjoy my family, and revel in the rest of my life with Claude.

Marion has had her fourth hernia repair, but the good news is she has remained cancer-free for several years. She continues to enjoy her large family and circle of friends.

Alice Cotter Feldman

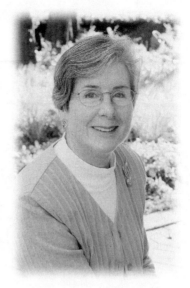

had a long, distinguished career in nursing after graduating from New York's Mt. Sinai Hospital School of Nursing. While raising five children, she returned to college, attending Pace University (New York), and graduated with honors at age forty-nine. Until her retirement, Alice hired and trained nursing staff personnel and developed policy procedure manuals. Well-published in a variety of medical journals, she also served as a guest adjunct professor at Columbia University in nursing education. Although her first marriage ended in divorce, Alice has been happily remarried for more than thirty-two years, blending her four children with her husband's only child. They are now the proud grandparents of nine. Today, Alice serves her community on local boards, participating in support groups and volunteering at a local hospital. Alice and her husband enjoy wintering at their home in the Florida Keys with family and friends.

DIAGNOSIS PROFILE

Age at diagnosis:	63 years old
Family history:	None
Symptoms:	Self-discovered lump
Surgery:	Core biopsy
	Lumpectomy
	Axillary node dissection
Biopsy results:	Infiltrating ductal carcinoma
	Stage: 2
	Tumor size: 1.8 cm.
	Nodes: 1 of 14 positive
	Estrogen and progesterone receptors positive
	Grade: 2
Chemotherapy:	Adriamycin/Cytoxan (AC)
Radiation therapy:	33 treatments
Hormonal therapy:	Tamoxifen
	Pre-diagnosis: 12 years of HRT

To each is given a bag of tools,
A shapeless mass, A book of rules;
And each must make, 'ere life is flown,
A stumbling block or a steppingstone.

—R. L. Sharpe

The Long Bald Summer

ALICE COTTER FELDMAN

It was a few days until the biggest celebration of my life: the millennium. I had been anticipating the year 2000 since I was a teenager. I was so excited to realize that I would, in fact, witness the event I had been fearful I would not live long enough to experience. Why? Because my family's medical history was filled with heart disease and vascular disease, taking most members of my father's family before the age of sixty.

My life, like so many others, has been filled with the "business of life" itself. Marriage, children, divorce, remarriage, work, college degrees earned as an adult, the children's educations, and then, their marriages and their children. It has been a full and, ultimately, satisfying life. My husband, Ron, and I were both sixty-two years old and were preparing for retirement. All of our children, four of mine from a first marriage and one of Ron's, were now grown, and four were married with children of their own.

Ron and I planned to leave cold, snowy New York and move

south to reap the rewards of our years of hard work. Throughout my life I have always been a planner, so why change now? Just before the move, I discovered that I had a heart problem—a faulty aortic valve. This defect had never been picked up during my physical exams and EKGs, which I had yearly due to my family's medical history. Nothing abnormal was ever found. But during a bout of pneumonia that winter, a heart murmur was detected. As a result of many tests, the diagnosis was a defective (bicuspid) aortic valve, with an ascending aortic aneurysm. The doctors warned me that the complications could be serious. I was told I would need to be reevaluated in six months and, oh yes, no heavy lifting in the meantime. This directive would prove to be the most difficult as we would soon have to pack up our thirteen-room house, hold three garage sales, put our house on the market, and say goodbye to all that we knew.

By the summer, we were on our way to taking permanent residence at our Florida house, a second home that we had rented out for almost ten years, while waiting for retirement. Our long-term plan was now a reality. Another part of the plan was to live in Georgia for six months of the year. One of our children had moved to Atlanta with his family, and we had visited them often, becoming familiar with the area and the wide range of services available. We also felt that the climate and the cost of living were favorable for us.

Once we were settled in our Florida home, we came up to Atlanta and found a small, lovely condo in a suburb north of the city. It was now time to start taking care of my medical needs. I searched out a cardiologist and went for my six-month evaluation. It was a surprise to learn that the findings showed increased thickening of the aortic valve with subsequent decrease in function. My only symptom was some shortness of breath, so I was taking it pretty easy. Along with the thickening valve was the strong possibility of a dissecting aneurysm, which could result in sudden death. I may have been looking for early retirement, but not that much retirement!

The decision was really made for me—I would have to undergo open-heart surgery for the placement of an artificial valve and the removal of the thinning aorta. The surgery would, of course, increase my total cardiac function. This surgery could very well have lengthened the lives of my relatives had it been available years ago.

Ron was more nervous than I was as we walked into the hospital before dawn for the scheduled 9:00 a.m. surgery. I wanted to allay his fears, so I said, "Everything will be fine; it's just a repair. My heart muscle is strong; all I need is a new part. After all, I don't have cancer or leukemia." Five months later those words would come back to haunt me.

The open-heart surgery and the need for a second open-heart surgery four days later, due to a complication, left me more debilitated than I had ever been in my life. I had always been a physically strong, athletic, and totally independent person. Now it was hard to breathe and difficult to walk from the bedroom to the living room in our small condo. My energy resource felt like a minus ten!

Along with the recuperation from the heart surgeries, I was suffering terribly from menopausal hot flashes. At the time of surgery I had to discontinue my hormone replacement therapy (HRT), and the dreaded symptoms immediately returned. I had taken HRT for twelve years because of the hot flashes, sleeplessness, and brain fog. Now they were all back. When I started HRT, I was working full time and I really needed relief in order to function. My gynecologist had prescribed it, and I had followed all the precautions, including annual mammograms and monthly self-examinations. All my queries regarding the safety of prolonged HRT were given a positive response, so I had no qualms about taking it.

Right after Christmas, I became very weepy. It had been the first holiday that we had not been surrounded by all the children and grandchildren at the old family homestead. We made a small attempt at holiday decorations, and it was just that—small. No tree, no lights, and in my depleted condition, I couldn't tell what made me the saddest: the condition of my body, now severely scarred, the total lack of physical strength, or the emotional loss of that beloved event—holidays with the whole family. Looking back, I'm sure it was a combination of all three. One month after heart surgery and after consultation with a menopause specialist and the cardiologist, it was decided that I could restart HRT. Hooray!

Every day I pushed myself to exercise—four minutes to six minutes to ten minutes to fifteen minutes, until I could walk thirty minutes at a time. I also used a portable breathing apparatus, known as an "incentive spirometer," four times a day to increase my lung capacity. There were some very low days, when I would go into the bathroom, turn on the shower, and sob. I didn't want Ron to know how dreadful I felt, and how I despaired of ever feeling like "Alice" again.

As I gained strength, my sense of humor returned and my normally positive attitude had found its way back. Also, thanks again to hormone replacement, I was sleeping better, and the hot flashes had diminished in number and intensity. Why, I was going to be just fine. Just as I planned.

At the end of January, Ron and I readied ourselves for our trip to Florida, where we would stay until June. We were already a month off the original timetable but needed to wait for my medical clearance in order to travel. We were both, once again, optimistic about the future. The cardiologist had given me the okay to resume normal activities, and I had initiated plans for cardiac rehab in Florida. All my medications appeared effective, with only slight concern about the medication Coumadin. Coumadin is a blood thinner required for patients with an artificial valve to prevent the formation of blood clots. Should a clot form and break away from the valve, it could cause a stroke or other organ disorders. Coumadin must be taken every day, and a blood test is done every two to four weeks until the correct therapeutic level is attained, with periodic blood tests thereafter. The other long-term effect of the heart surgery was the loud clicking sound from the artificial valve! At night, when all was quiet, Ron could hear the click-click-click. I got used to his asking me to turn over and change position to lessen the sound.

Ron had his annual physical exam the week prior to our planned departure, and we now waited for his final test results. As we were packing the car, the phone rang; it was Ron's internist. He cautioned Ron that his routine prostate serum analysis (PSA) was elevated and that he should follow up with a urologist ASAP. So we unpacked the car, made the necessary phone calls, and started on a new round of doctor visits, examinations, biopsies, a colonoscopy, an MRI, and a bone scan. The final verdict: prostate cancer. Immediate treatment was advised.

I am ashamed to admit that after the initial call about the elevated PSA, I was very disturbed and disappointed that all our plans would have to be put aside yet again. Then I realized how selfish of me. Ron had been at my side for the open-heart surgeries, and he encouraged me to exercise every day. He did all the cardiac stretches with me and walked with me in the mall when the weather was too cold to go outside. *Get over it, Alice; now it's time to be sure Ron is okay.*

Ron discussed all the options with his doctors and chose a course of external radiation, to be followed by the placement of radium seeds in the prostate. The radiation treatment would take place over five weeks, five days a week. The radium seeds implanted in the prostate would emanate radiation for two months, with specific precautions to be followed. The time span from the internist's initial call to the seed implantation was twelve weeks. With the seeds emanating radiation for two more months, the total time for Ron's treatment would be five months. Not exactly our idea of retirement.

As Ron went through his treatments, I went with him every day, and was also able to enroll in a cardiac rehab program at the hospital.

I went three times a week, which was a great boost to my physical and emotional self. I made friends with other cardiac patients and felt very lucky that my condition was corrected. My heart muscle was strong and healthy, with no clogged arteries. I was beating my family's odds.

During Ron's course of treatment and my rehabilitation, we had agreed to make the best of every day, so we took day trips in and around Atlanta. This was an opportunity to get to know the city and feel comfortable in it. We went to the theater, movies, museums, and joined a very active senior group. Though sometimes difficult to fit these excursions into our medical schedule, they somehow gave us a semblance of normalcy. After all, two serious and potentially life-threatening medical entities are trying on anyone or any relationship. When one of us is ill, both of us are affected, as well as our family and friends. Our mutual support of each other was, and continues to be, the foundation of our recovery. We accompanied each other to doctor visits and often had a special lunch date afterward. We were aware of the gift of time that we could give to each other because we were retired and were able to devote our full attention to the particular need of the day. How do people who work manage their lives through the emotional and physical roller coaster of serious illness? I can only marvel at their strength.

Cardiac rehab gave me renewed vigor and strength, and the HRT, once again, evened out my emotions. It was late March and we began to talk about going down to Florida after Ron's radium seed implant. Maybe we could get away by mid-April. We always liked the spring there, as the weather warmed and the days lengthened.

Uh-oh, what do I feel? As I showered, four days before Ron's radium seed implant, I felt a small lump in my right breast—the outer aspect. What is that? Is it hard? Is it moveable? Is it round or knobby? Oh my, why didn't I pay more attention to the numerous articles about breast cancer in the journals and magazines I had been reading in all the doctor's offices over the years? I had never worried about breast cancer. I had none of the risk factors and had been assured that the HRT taken for twelve years carried minimal risk. No female in my family had ever had cancer. When I browsed through magazines, I read articles on heart disease and would glibly turn the page when I came to an article on breast cancer; I was much more interested in the latest home-decorating trend. After all, I did my monthly breast self-exam and had annual mammograms. The risk factors did not apply to me. So then, why do I feel this grape-sized mass? And just when Ron is scheduled for his radiation seed implant in four days! Not fair.

As I thought about the possibility of cancer, I tried to remember my last self-exam. Oh yes, it was in mid-November before the open-heart surgery. But I had not done it recently, having been distracted by my recovery and by Ron's prostate cancer. I wasn't even doing a self-exam the day I found this—it was just *there*. How could this happen to us? Our third medical crisis in five months! I set aside my fears (could this be denial?) and decided not to tell Ron until after his surgery. He had enough to deal with. But I did make an emergency appointment with a gynecologist. A set of professional hands needed to feel the lump. Also, as anyone who is an organized planner knows, there would need to be referrals for further follow-up, insurance confirmations, etc., if necessary.

Ron's surgery went very well, and though he was quite sore, he was discharged late the same night. He had an indwelling foley catheter that made him feel and look ill as he moved about the house. We removed it on the second day and he felt better. It was then that I told him I was seeing the gynecologist and that I had found a lump in my right breast. I calmly reassured him it would probably be fine, but inside me was a nagging fear that I couldn't shake.

So it went like this:

April 12th: gynecological visit

April 13th: mammogram

April 16th: biopsy

April 19th: definitive diagnosis—infiltrating ductal carcinoma

April 21st: visit the surgeon

April 27th: admission to hospital

April 29th: lumpectomy with axillary node resection

Note: my early admission to the hospital was necessary to prepare for surgery, due to my intake of Coumadin.

Cancer, "the big C," is scary stuff. It is so unpredictable and elusive. Suppose it had spread to other parts of my body? How much surgery would I need? And was I going to die soon? There never seemed to be a definitive answer. The general response I heard over and over again was: everyone is different, everyone responds differently, and the percentages quoted are always plus or minus your given situation. Also, my years of nursing had given me an end-stage view of cancer with subsequent death, when indeed, there are many good years to be enjoyed from that initial diagnosis until death, whether from cancer or any other disease.

The day I had my mammogram was just awful. I went alone; Ron was not feeling well. I had a sense of doom and knew I just had to get through it. The receptionist and the nursing staff were calm and caring, but they could not alleviate my fears. As the technician moved from the first plate to the second plate, I felt as though I would fall to the floor. Standing at the mammography machine for the third plate was intolerable. I wanted to scream. I wanted to tear out of the room. I had flashbacks of my open-heart surgery. And now this. It was more than I could bear. I felt so stupid as I just stood there and bawled like a baby! The mammogram machine pulled painfully on the same chest muscles that had so recently been separated and sewn back together. The area around the lump was getting sore from the pressure, and my fear about the future was choking me.

Following the mammogram and an ultrasound, the radiology oncologist spoke to me gently and with compassion. She advised a biopsy immediately, which we scheduled for Friday, three days hence. What a long ride home that day! *Don't cry, keep your eyes on the road, hurry home and get a hug from Ron.*

He came with me the day of the biopsy. We were both very quiet, each one hoping against hope that the lump would be benign. After all, I had had a benign mass removed from my left breast twenty-five years earlier. We could be lucky again, couldn't we? "Hope is the thing with feathers/that perches in the soul," wrote Emily Dickinson.

While I was on the ultrasound table being prepared for the biopsy, I could see the lump on the screen, and it looked unassuming. Small, round, and well circumscribed. As the doctor took each biopsy punch, I could watch the screen and see the needle advance to the lump, pierce it, and pull back with the tissue to be examined. Three times, four times, five times total. In the end, the previously round, well-circumscribed lump was ragged on the lower edges, though still firm on top. As I looked at those ragged edges I was gripped with yet another fear. Suppose a cancer cell escapes into my bloodstream and travels to my brain or my liver or my pancreas. It could be there an indeterminate time and grow into a new cancer. Help! Conversation with the doctor allayed my immediate fears, and Ron and I came home to wait for the diagnosis from the laboratory. The doctor did inform us that a tumor the size of mine had been there at least eight years, which was shocking because it had not shown up on any of my prior mammograms.

Let's go to the telephone call that is forever burned in my memory. I was to get the biopsy results on a Tuesday, but the doctor called on Monday, in the early evening. I was in the bedroom and I took the call as I sat on the edge of the bed. When the doctor said the words *infiltrating ductal carcinoma*, with the need for immediate surgery, I became numb. I had thought it might be cancer but it was unspoken. Now the spoken words were clanging in my ears, and to me it was a death sentence. How was it possible? Not yet fully recovered from heart surgery and still caring for Ron, who needed to recuperate himself, I found this news cruel and unfair. In less than five months we were faced with *three* life-threatening crises—my anxiety was at an all-time high.

I went into the living room and told Ron. He was as shocked as I was. As we discussed the need to follow up and all the possible ramifications for our future, it occurred to me that in my preparation for open-heart surgery, I never felt anxiety. I had a strong heart with a defective valve. It would be replaced, I would heal, and there would be no lingering effects. (At that time I was not fully aware of the effects of Coumadin on future procedures and surgery.) I went into open-heart surgery without fear; I had complete faith in my surgeon and his team. I had even prepared for the surgery with relaxation tapes sent by a friend, and I had four relaxation sessions with personal tapes made for me; one for pre-surgery and one for post-surgery. They allowed me to turn over my relaxed body to my surgeon, in whom I had great trust. I even had the pre-surgical tape playing as I underwent anesthesia and used the post-surgical tape soon after I awakened. These tapes would surely come in handy again.

The news of *cancer* brought me to a whole new place—anxious, fearful, sad, angry, and depressed. As a person with usual equanimity, I now began to sway emotionally. Ron would find me crying at any time of the day or night. After the diagnosis on that fateful Monday night, I cried for two days. *Not me! Why me?*

Ron and I digested the information and started on a new journey, to remove the tumor and recover from breast cancer. We went off to the surgeon, off to the hospital, and off with part of my breast!

I was fortunate to need only a lumpectomy and an axillary node resection, though I had voluntarily signed for a full mastectomy, if needed. When I awoke from the surgery, I instinctively reached for my right breast and was relieved to have fared so well. This feeling of gratitude was confirmed when Ron, our son, and my sister met me with smiles of joy and relief.

Now we waited for the laboratory results regarding the tumor itself, i.e., margins, cell type, node involvement, etc. Most women go home the same day after a lumpectomy, but I had a nine-day stay due to Coumadin. I was admitted to the hospital two days prior to surgery to be "heparinized" for the surgery, i.e., placed on a continuous IV of Heparin, and taken off Coumadin. Heparin is a fast-acting anticoagulant, which the doctors can manipulate very quickly in an emergency. After the lumpectomy, it took seven days for my blood to return to acceptable levels so I could be discharged from the hospital.

The symptoms of menopause started to plague me again. I had stopped HRT as soon as the cancer was suspected. It was now early May and the hot flashes, sleeplessness, and the dullness of my brain returned. I describe the dullness of my brain this way: a cloud descends over my head and rests on my shoulders. I see everything around me as dulled, and I am slow on the uptake and response. No matter how hard I try to duck my head down to get out from under the cloud, it doesn't work. Therefore, all experiences are from the vantage point of gray.

The laboratory results were finally in. It was Stage 2 carcinoma with clean margins, estrogen and progesterone positive with minor lymph node involvement. The surgeon's report was somewhat upbeat as he discussed further treatment options and, along with the oncologist, we decided to pursue chemotherapy and radiation, followed by five years of tamoxifen. It all sounded cut-and-dried when, in fact, it was actually quite difficult to concentrate on the information as the depth of the problems we faced began to sink in.

I tried to put on a happy face for day-to-day living. In past adversities I had always looked for some good in the situation and was able to maintain a positive attitude. This, of course, is great for those around you, but it did not serve *me* well. There were many unresolved sadnesses from the past that surfaced when the surgery was over and the treatments for cancer progressed. They needed attention, and I needed to pay attention.

We could not go to Florida; we continued to be confined by illness, and I joined the thousands of other women in chemo and radiation with all the possible complications ahead. Ron and I were becoming a boring couple. All we could talk about was our last treatment or treatments to come—not exactly cocktail-hour conversation.

Before the surgery there was the issue of whether to notify family and friends. How can I describe the calls to our five children, other family members and friends, to inform them of this latest crisis? Can it be put in soft tones or gentle words? How difficult to allay their fears over the phone. Should we even *tell* them? After all, they have their own full lives, their families, and careers. In the end, we decided that the truth was necessary. These were difficult conversations as we heard the pain and concern of those we love. Subsequently, I feel a large part of my recovery was directly due to the overwhelming support, prayers, and love of everyone we told. My sisters, who lived in Key West, sent Reiki (a form of meditation which seeks to restore order to the body whose vital energy has become unbalanced) "across the miles," neighbors placed me in their ongoing prayer groups and brought dinners, and we received a steady stream of calls from so many. Each note, phone call, visit, e-mail, and other acts of kindness would be forever recorded in my heart.

Once the trauma of telling all those who needed to know was over, it was back to the planning stage. We made a quick trip to

Florida for business reasons, then a trip to New York to see the rest of the family before I started chemotherapy. The physicians gave the okay for the trips, which were satisfying and strengthened my resolve to recover completely.

When I got back to Atlanta, I met again with the oncologist to finalize the course of action. A port-a-cath would be placed in my chest wall, below the clavicle, so that the chemotherapeutic agents would be delivered through the port directly into my bloodstream. Without the port, veins in the arm are used and there is the danger that they can be compromised. As with all breast-cancer surgery where lymph nodes are removed, the affected side needs to be protected from future blood drawing and blood pressure checks. It is to be protected as much as possible from cuts, abrasions, and burns. The port-a-cath was placed after I stopped my Coumadin, and I had to give myself a series of painful injections, which I vowed I would never do again. These injections were in place of Heparin, and I took them at home, thus avoiding hospitalization.

It was decided that my tumor type would respond well to a treatment of four infusions of Adriamycin and Cytoxin. Each infusion would be three weeks from the first and/or preceding infusion. Following the chemo, there would be six and a half weeks of radiation. By my calculations, the treatments would be completed in early November. What a long summer ahead!

In mid-June, I had my first chemo treatment. Ron and I drove to the Georgia Cancer Specialists treatment center with heavy hearts, each of us trying to put up a good front. Before the chemo was started, I received the medications Decadron and Kytril to decrease the chance of nausea. Though I was somewhat apprehensive, the first treatment went very well. The nursing staff was outstanding and anticipated my needs so that my anxiety levels were lessened. I was fortunate to receive treatment in a cancer center, a large room edged with recliner chairs where the nurses had full visibility of the patients at all times. The latest magazines were there, as well as refreshments (if tolerated). Common bonds were struck between the patients who were receiving chemo.

Two hours later we were on our way home, and I was pleased that there was no nausea thus far, and I was actually hungry. In fact, the only immediate side effect I experienced from the first chemo was absolute sleeplessness—I stayed awake for thirty-nine hours! Apparently, I had a reaction to the Decadron and was assured the dosage would be decreased in the future. I continued to take the anti-nausea drugs, and except for a flushing in my face and the sleeplessness of menopause, I felt okay. Not great, but okay.

I was aware that my hair would fall out from the chemo, and other chemo patients said it should take two weeks after the first treatment to start coming out. Prior to my cancer, I had seen many women in wigs, turbans, and scarves. Each time I felt a twinge of discomfort for them. Soon it would be me.

Here are some excerpts from the journal I kept during the course of chemotherapy:

June 24th. Had blood work done and my counts are down. I was cautioned to stay out of crowds and not to eat fresh fruits and salads. This is called neutropenic precautions.

June 27th. Again today I feel very good. Full of energy (psychic) and happy. I seem to be on a new plane. I feel I have finally accepted the cancer diagnosis, and with all the treatments and the love and support of family and friends, it will be okay—successful for the eradication of cancer cells in my body. I feel calm and centered and seem to have maintained my sense of humor. My hair is looking particularly good as I prepare to lose it. A new shampoo and a little longer length have made my hair a bit wavy and soft.

June 29th. Had another blood count done yesterday and it shows the WBC and granulocytes very low, leaving me open for an overwhelming infection. Should I get an infection of any kind, with chills and fever, I need to get to a hospital immediately. At this point, Ron and I cancel a three-day trip to Virginia. My hair is still there but my scalp is sore, it tingles. Maybe this is the beginning.

July 2nd. As expected, my hair started to come out two days ago. Slowly at first, and my scalp was sore. Yesterday the hair loss increased, and today my scalp is clearly visible. I have been up since 5:00 a.m. and feel sad today. I think the hair loss makes such a visible statement. Before, I could go out and no one knew I had cancer. Now, just to look at me is to know it. This hair loss needs to be grieved just as other losses are. I am not too good at giving myself the time to grieve, at least not until now. But, ironically, our life's pace has slowed. I can now consciously deal with the pain of loss. Ron is very sweet and supportive as my hair comes out. I can just pull it gently and out it comes! At this point, it will look better all out. We may shave it, if it looks like it would be best.

July 4th. I shed a few tears as my hair was coming out. Once I'd lost enough to need a covering for my head, it somehow became easier to look at, and I make every effort to cover my head as attractively as possible. So we've come to another milestone—may God protect us from what's to come and may a cure be possible.

July 6th. Hooray, today my blood counts had improved and I was able to get the second chemo. Decadron was decreased by half so that I did not experience the sleeplessness as before. I also was given a sleeping pill, which was a great help. Again, following treatment, my face flushed bright red and that lasted two days.

July 9th. Had an appointment with the nutritionist. She cautions me to cut back on my food portions due to my weight gain (six pounds). It is surprising that many women, myself included, gain weight while on chemotherapy. Isn't that ironic? The average weight gain is thirteen pounds I am told, and I am moving in that direction quickly. It seems our appetites increase, whether physical or emotional elements are at work. In any case, at a certain point, it becomes a concern. For myself, I was eating whatever I wanted, which is not my usual style. I had been careful about food intake for years, since age sixteen!

July 15th. I awoke very subdued and was weepy all day. The tears would flow easily, and I seemed to have no control over them. Ron tries to console me, but to no avail. At bedtime, it is worse. I really miss the person I used to be, strong and healthy. At this time, I feel I've been sick a long time and November seems so far away. I really miss the children and their families. So much seems to be passing me by. I am praying every night for strength to graciously get through this time, and having no hair is no help! I follow Oprah's suggestion to enumerate six items from the day to be grateful for, and it has been helpful.

The weather has been hot, so a scarf and a cap to cover my head are hotter! The hot flashes are stronger after the chemo (second), but no nausea. Last night I was having a pity party. My right breast, the surgical side, has been hurting for two days. As I roll on my right side it hurts, on the left side my port-a-cath hurts, my mid-chest is all scarred and my heart is always noisy—click, click, click. And my head is bare. I sure have changed in six months.

The days moved on uneventfully and we were kept busy with our new computer, our first. I worked on my needlepoint, Ron and I did all the household chores, food shopping, etc. One day ran into the next as we counted down to the third chemo. I had purchased a wig but did not like it. It made me look like The Church Lady from

Saturday Night Live. I felt sharper and more attractive in the scarves, hats, and baseball caps, of all color combinations, to match my clothes. I continued on neutropenic precautions—no crowds, no fresh fruits or vegetables. I carried an antibacterial hand sanitizer to cleanse my hands after touching areas in public use, and I carried my own pen to sign credit card receipts. These were small, but comforting, precautions.

Ron continued to be a source of strength. His radiation treatments were over and he had become stronger. He wrote me love notes, and told me I was pretty every day. He was always boosting my femininity. One night as I readied myself for bed, I walked into the bedroom and Ron was sitting cross-legged on the bed with a scarf on his head. He said, "If you wear a scarf, I will wear a scarf!" It cracked me up. We also had a conversation about how important a clean house was to me at this time. We had a cat and it was necessary to vacuum often, as I felt it was important to protect my immune system from outside assault. Ron cooperated in all these requests, and I was so grateful.

During this time we were fortunate to have visits from our Atlanta family, our daughters from New York, and old friends who stayed a few days on their way through Atlanta. Two of my sisters and Ron's brother came as well, and every visit was a boost.

My third chemo treatment was postponed—again my blood count was too low. This was a disappointment, but two days later everything was back on track. We left the Georgia Cancer Specialists early in the afternoon and, once home, I felt uneasy. I wasn't hungry for a change. Instead, I became violently ill, vomiting and retching for another seven hours. Ron contacted the doctor and went to the pharmacy for more anti-nausea medication. Though I felt awful that night, I knew how lucky I was. Some patients feel that terrible most of the time. I couldn't imagine.

Again from my journal:

    During the time of continued vomiting and rushing to the
bathroom, I could not keep my nightcap on. Once I lost my hair,
I purchased a lacy nightcap to wear as I prepared for bed and for
first thing in the morning. It helped me to feel better about
myself, and I hoped it would make me a bit more attractive. But,
during this siege I couldn't keep the nightcap on, and Ron got a
clear view of my noble dome! He took great care of me, putting
cool cloths to my forehead and kissing my head. All through the
night I alternated between having the chills (under two blankets)
and throwing off the covers with the heat and perspiration of hot
flashes. Can't say I feel too romantic these days.

    It may sound corny, but during this time, I offered up all my
discomforts for the families of the people shot by Mark Barton.
He had recently killed twelve people and wounded thirteen in
Atlanta. How does a person get so desperate? My illness is very
small next to the pain of those victims and their families.

Due to the low blood counts after the first two chemos, I now
had to take injections every day for ten days after the third chemo.
This medication, Neupogen, helps the body restore the cells compromised by the treatments. I essentially felt okay for the remainder
of the treatment course, if you consider sleeplessness, hot flashes,
and general malaise okay. We were able to take rides in the country,
enjoy lunch dates, watch videos, see the grandchildren, attend support groups, attend the symphony, participate in a book group, etc.
It was important to us to make every day count and to be proactive
to that end.

The sleepless nights had a positive side (I can say this now). All
my life I had been blessed with the ability to sleep well. I would fall
asleep the moment my head hit the pillow, and always slept a solid
seven to eight hours a night. Now, after lying awake for hours, night

after night, I came to know why great inventions and plots for best-sellers are conjured up in the middle of the night. One has ample time to write a trilogy.

Nighttime became my time to reminisce: to reconstruct child-hood, to recall the wonderful experience of having children, and evaluate the course my life had taken. It was a time to sort out sad-nesses, losses, guilts, but also to acknowledge accomplishments. Surprisingly, for me, I returned to prayer after years of ignoring this aspect of my life. It took me over a week to reconstruct the formal prayers of my childhood. Chemotherapy patients experience a change in mental capacity; we jokingly call it "chemo brain." Thus, I credited chemo brain for my inability to easily call up the rituals of the past. But, I again found comfort in prayer and also enjoyed con-versations with God and with deceased family members. No, they did not answer me, but I felt calmer after experiencing concentrated memories of those loved ones and admitting to them (and myself) my shortcomings, and how I could have handled some past situa-tions differently. A lot of self-awareness, not always comfortable, was reckoned with and reconciled. To me, therein lies the answer. For so many years, the business of daily living and the sound sleep at night did not allow time for self-reflection. Here was the opportunity to do so, and I seized it.

My journal has a long entry where I recalled the summers of my youth. Carefree days at the beach, sailing all summer with friends, family picnic breakfasts, fireworks—all were rich in my memory and the details surprised me. I recalled the physical layout of a beach club our family enjoyed, each building, beach, ramp, and barbecue area. Why, I could actually smell the salty air as my mind lingered on the swimming races and the sailing regattas that domi-nated my early years.

It was also during those long nights that the old issues of aban-donment and loss reentered my consciousness. Why had it taken so long to think about it? Was it all too painful to address in the day-time when ordinary living crowded out the emotional issues? Whatever—now I could recall and revisit those issues and work through them, many times becoming so emotional I'd have to get out of bed so as not to disturb Ron. I was also working through the move away from my family in New York; my role as a mother and grandmother was being redefined, at least geographically, and set-tling into a new community took energy. When I first discovered I would be fighting cancer, I felt abandoned by God—at that time we were not on great terms—and then subsequently experienced a great loss of self due to the surgery and chemotherapy's side effects. Now it became easier to explore all the wounds and, hopefully, heal them. After all, when the treatments were over, there was a long, produc-tive life to continue living.

On a hot day in August, Friday the 13th to be exact, we were returning home from a shopping trip only to be rear-ended at a stop-light. When we were hit, our heads lurched backward against the headrests and then forward. My scarf and hat flew off my head and into the back seat! The man who had accidentally hit us jumped out of his car, ran to us, and as he peered into our car, a look of fear came over his face. He was staring past Ron at me and I could hear him thinking, "What have I done? This woman has lost her hair!—all I did was hit their bumper." As I retrieved my hat and scarf, we reas-sured him he was not responsible for my baldness. Then came the usual exchange of insurance information, registration, etc. On the way home, I reminded Ron it was Friday the 13th, and we both started laughing.

On to the fourth and last chemo treatment at the end of August. During that time, my sister visited from Florida and our daughter came down from New York. Each visit was precious and lessened the effects of the chemo. Again, I gave myself Neupogen shots for ten days, and I must say I was getting "gun-shy." I felt my body had been assaulted enough. My appetite was minimal and my mind dull. My balance was off and I was very quiet. The bad taste in my mouth was continuous, and I was sure I *smelled* of chemo when I perspired, which was often due to the hot flashes, day and night.

Labor Day weekend arrived, and spending the holiday without my beloved family gatherings made me feel homesick. Sometimes when I was sad or discouraged, I would say to myself, "I want to go home." But where was home? Which home was I looking for? My childhood home where Mom took care of me? My home in New York where all the children grew into such wonderful adults? My home in Florida where the waters of the Gulf outside my windows soothed my soul and the sun warmed my bones? The answer I came to was: to have inner peace and stay "in the moment"—that's home. Enjoy the present, for in truth, it is all we have. *So, get real Alice, and get on with it,* I scolded myself. The way it was is not going to be again. Not just in celebrating holidays, but in my place in family life, as well as personal issues that affected Ron and me. Our serious medical conditions changed how we lived our daily lives. Our relationship deepened, yet our expectations of each other lessened. It was complicated, and we often talked about our "realignment of life."

We spent early September glued to the TV, watching the U.S. Open and rooting excitedly for Andre Agassi. The following week I had to prepare for radiation. The preparation, called a "simulation," created the head and neck mold that would be used in every treatment thereafter to keep my body in alignment during the treatments. As the mold was setting, technicians made mathematical calculations and set coordinates for the radiation beams, which had to perfectly match up to the markings on my breast made by the radiation oncologist. As I dressed and undressed, I couldn't help but look at my body. There were the visible scars, but there were also many invisible ones. In the still, softly lit room, the four technicians worked quietly, clarifying their numerical findings with one another. It was just routine for them, but for me it was another confirmation of the severity of the cancer diagnosis—my mortality rose up again and was choking me. As I lay on the table and the staff worked quietly around me, I hoped no one would notice the tears dropping off my cheeks onto the new, plastic mold.

The transition from chemotherapy to radiation went smoothly. Six days after the simulation and three weeks after the last chemo, my daily course of radiation started. There would be thirty-three treatments, twenty-eight regular and five "booster," over a six-and-a-half week period. All along the treatment course, I had been very proactive in making appointments with the doctors for every required test and treatment. I felt that to do otherwise would have resulted in a loss of time, and our plans would be put on hold. We had decided to go to New York for Thanksgiving, and I didn't want any avoidable delay to interfere with that. We had canceled too many plans due to treatment postponements and side effects. I was determined to be ready for this trip.

The course of radiation was uneventful. I was there every day at 8:30 a.m., and the treatment itself took no more than five to eight minutes. It took me longer to undress and dress, with the added attention to my scarf and hat, than to get the radiation. The staff was friendly and cheerful every day. I would lie on a movable table with my head and neck in my mold and my right (affected) arm raised over my head holding on to a bar. My scarred and marked breast was exposed, the table moved into position and the machine's beams were coordinated for my specific needs. Then the staff left the room, cautioning me not to move. The patient's body position is observed on TV monitors, and then they turn on the radiation. The room is dim and there is a low buzzing sound, which I always tried to count out but reached a different number every day.

Fortunately, my skin did not burn or blister with radiation. My sister had sent me a cream that was 98 percent aloe, and I applied it liberally twice a day. Some women use the aloe plant itself with good results. If necessary, prescription medication is available. I also did not experience the fatigue so often associated with radiation. So, once the treatment was completed in the morning, the rest of our day was free. We managed to fill the days constructively and take in special events. Ron and I attended an art class for watercolor instruction, which was a first for us. It opened my mind to the many possibilities for future adventures. We took computer classes twice a week. Now the days passed quickly. We were also active in condo committees and in our respective cancer support groups.

I truly believe that support groups are invaluable for the breast-cancer patient. It is so important to get as much information as possible from the women who have walked the same road. Women bond easily and under the common threat of cancer, bonding is practically immediate. A sisterhood is formed, information flows freely, and advice from those sisters further along the treatment course is priceless.

Since the women brought the best advice of their doctors to each meeting, the pooled information educated us all. Physical problems are candidly discussed. Usually someone in the group has experienced the same problem or knows someone who has. Emotional issues are numerous. The varied emotions of the patients themselves as they deal with work problems, family matters, body image, etc., all require airing. Family structures suffer as roles change; often women share the mixed reactions regarding their husbands, their parents, and their teenage daughters. A good support group is a safe place to verbalize concerns without censure. Love, empathy, and total support help many through these difficult days.

I originally attended two separate groups and discovered that an all-female group accomplished the most. When the group is mixed (male and female), some subjects do not surface for the obvious reason: the participants are shy and reticent to discuss personal issues.

I left the mixed group after five weeks. The female breast-cancer group met monthly and seemed to draw out those who had the greatest need. Then everyone would rally around those particular women. Good leadership is necessary to keep any group alive. There were so many small but helpful hints we could provide one another, i.e., purchasing a special toothpaste for the dry mouth that comes with chemo, shampoos specially formulated for hair that is growing back, and makeup tricks for the loss of eyelashes and eyebrows. We discussed medications for specific symptoms, and I was then able to ask my doctor about prescribing them for me. We talked about foods and diets, juicing, alternative modalities, and physical therapy for regaining muscle function and for the complication of lymphedema. The list is endless.

In late September, I started on tamoxifen, the oral chemotherapeutic medication that was prescribed once a day for five years. Since I still complained of hot flashes, the oncologist prescribed an additional chemotherapeutic agent, Megace, which would decrease the number and severity of the hot flashes. Four weeks later, the flashes subsided substantially and I could sleep much better. What joy and relief. The sense that I exuded a chemo odor diminished and eventually went away altogether.

Then I received a nice reward. I was chosen to represent my hospital's support group to be a model in a "Pink Ribbons" fashion show to be held in October, for Breast Cancer Awareness Month, at an exclusive downtown hotel. The month of October was filled with luncheons, walks, runs, and special events to raise public awareness of the need for funding and research to find the cure for this disease. I listened to, and had the privilege to meet, Dr. Susan Love, author of *Dr. Susan Love's Breast Book*, as well as the late Susan Sturges-Hyde, author of *No More Bad Hair Days*.

At the fashion show, I was the only survivor to wear a headscarf; the others either had grown their hair back or wore attractive wigs. I felt that my wig was not the most flattering—the makeup/hair artist agreed. So I walked the runway in an elegant black evening pantsuit, beautiful shoes and jewelry supplied by an upscale department store, and my humble scarf. It was great!

Radiation treatments ended in late October, and we were right on schedule. Now the only procedure remaining was the removal of the port-a-cath. During the last weeks of radiation, I met with my surgeon and cardiologist to plan for the removal. I was in the hospital five days for a procedure that typically takes twenty minutes with a stay of two to three hours. I had to be hospitalized for five full days: two days with a heparin drip, on day three the port removal, and then two more days of heparin drip and the restart of Coumadin. I decided to make my stay productive. I addressed our Christmas cards, read two books, and worked on my needlepoint. I also found that my hospital stays were far more tolerable when I took my own clothes to wear during the day. I dressed in lightweight slacks, T-shirts, and comfortable shoes. This confused the staff who kept asking, "Where is the patient?" I loved that little feeling of control that it gave me.

Peace of mind is truly a blessing, and I was fortunate to have it during this hospitalization. I was calm and, in fact, somewhat exuberant. After all, this was the last procedure in a process that had started seven and a half months earlier. By this time, Ron's PSA was down to within normal limits and he was feeling strong. So was I, a little bit more each day. I was sleeping again and beginning to see the positive side of any situation. I had grown stronger, thanks to the strength and love of those around me.

It was at this time that another survivor introduced me to the breast-cancer support group at The Wellness Community. They met weekly and provided another forum for mutual respect and support. I found the group's dynamics differed each week. There was so much support through multiple services such as nutrition, stress reduction, caregiver groups, massage, art therapy, and on and on. The group was open, caring and loving, and the sessions were run with the full understanding of the participants' needs, whether a survivor or a caregiver.

Now it was on to New York for a three-week visit. My hair was growing in, and there were times when I could go without a hat. More joy. Being with family and friends made Thanksgiving truly worth giving thanks for. I felt overwhelming gratitude to have the children, their spouses, and grandchildren all around a festive holiday table.

So, as I waited for the millennium and the celebrations to begin, I wondered how I would recall the past year as we moved into the twenty-first century. It had been a year of three medical crises, multitudinous doctor visits, many hospital stays, and lengthy treatments. We experienced numerous physical and emotional changes. And I was bald, all over. And yet, it was also a year of great personal growth and wisdom, and an increased ability to accept, unconditionally, the love and support of family and friends.

For me, the side effects of Coumadin will be everlasting, but the effects of the chemotherapy had their positive side. My hair grew back darker and very curly, my complexion improved, my mouth felt cleaner with decreased tartar, and my nails were stronger. My appetite was huge—I could eat the patterns off the plates! Although my weight was up, I felt great—I just bought clothes with elastic waistbands.

I learned that all planning is for naught when our health is at stake, and all plans are flexible. The diagnosis of cancer is not an automatic death sentence, and it is beneficial to work through our life issues so that peace of mind frees us up to heal.

I gained in unexpected ways. I found the sisterhood of the support groups and recaptured the comfort of prayer. Gratitude for the abundance of daily gifts, no matter how simple, enriches my life. My relationship with Ron deepened as we realigned our daily living needs and/or limitations of any given situation.

The old adage "every day is precious" took on new meaning. We would be diligent with our attention to our bodies' changes, and I promised to continue breast self-exams. We vowed to love, support, and nurture our family and friends, hoping to give back a small measure of what we received from them.

And so, on millennium eve, I cheerfully shouted, "Come on year 2000 and beyond—we are ready!"

Since my treatments ended, I have gone through many changes. Physically I feel fine, even as I struggle with Coumadin swings. My weight is still up but has leveled off, my hair has straightened out, and I walk two to three miles, five days a week.

Ron and I spend the winter in our home in the Florida Keys. We make frequent visits back to New York and Connecticut to stay connected to our family and friends there and, joyfully, we have set down roots in our new community in a suburb of Atlanta. We volunteer at our local hospital, our senior center, and our church, which we joined a year ago. We continue to take watercolor painting classes and are active on our condo committees. We support the many walks and benefits for the research and cure for cancer, and stay active in our support groups, more to give than to receive. I was elected to the executive board of The Cancer Survivors' Network of St. Joseph's Hospital. All these activities afford us the opportunity to give back to our community and to strengthen our network.

Finally, I see people I know in the grocery store and at the mall. . . . It feels like home.

Alice recently underwent a hysterectomy—the results were benign— but complications required a second surgery. Alice is recovering and planning to resume her full and busy life. Her cancer is still in remission.

Elena Tillán Santamaria

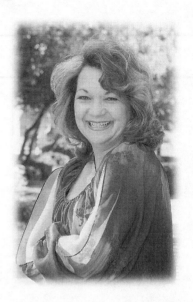

was born in Cuba and moved to Miami, Florida, at the age of five. She has completed two years toward a bachelor's degree in Health Administration and works as Lead Patient Advocate at Northside Hospital in Atlanta. Elena sees to the special needs of the patients and their visitors, offers cancer patients hope, and serves as a Spanish inter- preter. She attends health fairs and reaches out to both English- and Spanish-speaking women by talking with them about the importance of early detection and self breast exams. When not working, she enjoys dancing, hiking, jazzercise, reading, swimming, and yoga. Elena has two children and two young grandsons.

DIAGNOSIS PROFILE

Age at diagnosis:	46 years old
Family history:	Paternal aunt, three female cousins
Symptoms:	None—abnormal mammogram
Surgery:	Stereotactic core biopsy
	Mastectomy
	TRAM flap reconstruction
Biopsy results:	Infiltrating ductal carcinoma
	Stage: 2
	Tumor size: 2.4 cm
	Nodes: 7 negative
	Grade: 3
	Estrogen receptor negative
	S phase: 24.8%
Chemotherapy:	Adriamycin/Cytoxan (AC)
Hormonal therapy:	None

*Even when our life is most difficult, it is important
to remember that something within us is keeping us alive—
the life force—that lifts us, energizes us, pulls us back
sometimes from the abyss of despair.*
—Nathaniel Branden, Ph.D.

Tears of Triumph

ELENA TILLÁN SANTAMARIA

August 2001, Washington, D.C.
My voice trembled and my eyes were teary as I addressed the scientists. "On behalf of all breast-cancer survivors, I want to thank you for your dedication in the past and your continued drive and urgency in finding a cure. You are our hope!" One of the scientists quickly stood up. "We may be your hope, but *you* are our inspiration." Thus ended three wonderful, very challenging days of evaluating and voting on research proposals at the annual U.S. Department of Defense Breast-Cancer Research meeting in Washington, D.C.

A few months earlier, when I had been nominated to participate in this important meeting, I was not only flattered and excited, but realized it was an opportunity to expand my role as an advocate for patients and their families at Northside Hospital in Atlanta, Georgia. The timing of this invitation was also serendipitous: it was received on the second-year anniversary of my completion of chemotherapy.

Being asked to participate at this special conference would also reinforce the goal of helping scientists to better understand the human side of their research, and allow for funding decisions that would reflect the concerns and needs of breast-cancer patients.

After my own breast-cancer diagnosis, mastectomy, breast reconstruction, and treatment—the disease stopped my life for a year—I promised myself I would come out of this and would help others diagnosed with cancer. I now had a mission.

I know how much it means to a breast-cancer patient to meet a survivor—to see someone who is healthy, productive, working, and has been through what they're about to go through. I know what they are feeling deep inside, and just making that connection with them is so encouraging and hopeful for the patient, and so rewarding for me. I share my own battle stories and feel blessed that, in some ways, I am able to make a difference in this war on cancer.

Only two years earlier, I was wearing a wig to cover my bald head and flying down to Florida to visit my son and make plans for his wedding's dress rehearsal dinner. I arrived at Hartsfield International Airport still coping with the side effects of my chemotherapy, feeling weak, achy, and very tired. My blood count was too low, and I shouldn't have been traveling. But I had to prove to myself that I could make the trip and help my son plan his wedding.

Now here I was, dashing through the airport again, feeling like my old self, strong and healthy, my hair grown back, thicker and full of curls. My journey through breast cancer had become an empowering event in my life, and my experience with cancer itself was more that of a friend than an enemy. My discouragement had turned into encouragement, my bitterness into forgiveness. My adversity became my new strength.

And now I was going to tell that to the nation's top scientists at their research meeting in Washington, D.C.

* * * * *

I am a daughter, wife, mother, grandmother, friend, and patient advocate. I am also a breast-cancer survivor. Every one of my roles has deeply fulfilled me and shaped who I am. If you are someone who is just beginning the battle with breast cancer, feeling the fear and worry, enduring the rigorous treatments, it may be hard for you to believe this right now. If you have finished the treatments and are now picking up where your life left off before you were diagnosed with cancer, you will know exactly what I mean. Life *is* much sweeter now.

Being a cancer survivor has brought me to a place where I have a new sense of inner peace and strength. I savor all the special moments that life offers. I love more deeply. I am a stronger and more confident woman now. In Spanish we say: *"Lo que no te mata, te hace mas fuerte."* (If you can pull through the worst, you come out stronger and wiser when it's over.) Of course, all the confidence and wisdom I now possess is the opposite of what I felt when I first heard the words every woman fears: *You have breast cancer.*

From the moment I received my diagnosis, I felt like a failure to Bert, my husband of twenty-five years. I felt I had also failed my two grown children, Jaclyn and Dan. Because by having to tell them this scary news, I was going to bring them so much pain at what was supposed to be the highest, most joyful point in their lives. The emotions I went through—fear, sadness, worry, anger, powerlessness, and the incredible guilt—were overwhelming.

My life, especially the year before my diagnosis, was filled with a great deal of activity and, of course, not an inkling of the adversity that awaited me. On a very hot, typically beautiful June day in Savannah, Georgia, I stood looking at the huge, white wedding tent in Forsyth Park, adorned with dozens of flowers, near the exquisite fountain that resembles the one in the Place de la Concorde in Paris. After months of planning, the big day had finally arrived—our daughter's wedding. So many family members and good friends were arriving from out of town. The wedding was being held at the park, and the reception was indoors, in a hotel along the historic Riverfront.

I had a very special honor at Jaclyn's wedding. I was her matron of honor. Months earlier she had said to me, "Mom, you have always been there for me. You are not only my mom, you are also my best friend."

Throughout the years, due to Bert's job, we had moved a great deal. It was always hard to say goodbye to our good friends and start over again in a new city and state. But I think all this moving made my relationship with Jaclyn closer, because we spent a lot of time together. We took aerobics classes, attended history class at the university, and I never missed one of her dance recitals. I remember how upset she was when she started a new high school in Savannah. She missed her friends back home. I would try to cheer her up by playing and dancing to "I Will Survive." Since we both love to dance, the upbeat music and inspirational lyrics would pull her out of the doldrums. How ironic that I would be playing the song again, only this time for me.

Cancer is not new to my family. Both my father and Bert's mother had died from it. Bert's mother, in spite of her condition, strived to make it to Jaclyn's wedding. We were so grateful and honored that all of the grandparents traveled far to celebrate this very special day. However, we were not sure, until the last minute, if my mother-in-law, Elsa, would make it. In fact, she had been given only three months to live just prior to Jaclyn's wedding. But her incredibly strong will prevailed, and she got to see her granddaughter happily married. My own father had lost his battle with throat cancer fourteen years earlier, but he was with us in spirit that day. I was blessed to have my mother there to share in the happy occasion.

Jaclyn was radiant and lovely, and Bert was so elegant and proud as he walked her down the aisle. Our son, Danny, was also in the wedding party. Tall and handsome, and very much the young man on the move, with big dreams and big plans. He had just landed a good job in Boca Raton, Florida, and had also recently met a wonderful young woman.

As I watched both my grown children that day, I felt overwhelming joy and pride at who they had become. When they were young, I postponed my career to focus on raising them. I remembered their trusting eyes, first steps, first words, their tender touch, their hugs, and their *besitos* (kisses). God had given me two precious gifts who grew into caring, responsible, wonderful people.

One major life event comes to a close, and another one begins. The week after the wedding, I started preparing for our fourth move. Again, due to his job, for the previous year, Bert had been living in Atlanta, away from me. He was waiting for me to finish the wedding preparations, so we had been taking turns commuting on the weekends between Atlanta and Savannah. This would be our fourth time starting completely over. Our fourth time selling the house, finding a new one, finding a new job, making new friends, finding new doctors—everything. But this move would even be more difficult because we would have to say goodbye to Jaclyn and our new son-in-law, Chris. I told myself, my kids are happy; time to let go and start a new life. Besides, our twenty-fifth wedding anniversary was coming up in six months, and Bert and I were planning to spend it in Hawaii.

To say that life in Atlanta started on a stressful note would be an understatement. One month after the wedding, we received the sad news that my mother-in-law had passed away. A short time later, I was involved in an automobile accident—a car ran a red light and broadsided my vehicle. The impact was severe and I was rushed to the hospital. Fortunately, there was no major trauma and no broken bones, but I was left with neck and shoulder pain and had to begin physical therapy. Then, a few weeks prior to closing on the sale of our Savannah home, a storm snapped a tree, causing it to fall through the roof. We hadn't yet found a new home in Atlanta, and I was still looking for a new job.

Finally, things started to settle down, or so I thought. I had been offered a position as a patient advocate at Northside Hospital. I would be handling concerns from patients, family members, and visitors, plus providing encouragement and support to them. I had no idea how significant and instrumental my place of work would be in my impending battle.

We eventually found a lovely two-story home. The day we made our offer on the house, I received a reminder letter from my physician in Savannah that my yearly mammogram was several months overdue. I had completely forgotten about it with everything else that was happening, which is really not like me—I take things like that seriously.

When I was seventeen years old, while showering, I had felt a lump in my breast. Luckily, it turned out to be benign. Of course it is rare, but there have been cases of teenagers diagnosed with breast cancer. I was diagnosed with fibrocystic breast disease, and since then had always kept a close eye on my health, getting checked regularly. Then, during the past two years, prior to our move to Atlanta, I had felt a few lumps that turned out to be benign, liquid-filled cysts. These were aspirated with a needle. As simple as that. But it was now definitely time to have that overdue mammogram.

At Northside, I asked a coworker to recommend a doctor, and I made an appointment for a complete physical, including a Pap smear. When the examination was over, I left with two referrals: one for a mammogram and the other for an ultrasound of my uterus. (For many years, I have been watched closely for a benign fibroid in my uterus.) As the technician was performing my pelvic ultrasound, I asked her if she could check to see if perhaps there had been a cancellation, so that I could have my mammogram done that same day. My scheduled appointment was for two weeks later, but my instincts were telling me to have it done now—I don't know why, but it suddenly felt urgent. *Que alivio!* I was relieved and thankful when this technician, a wonderful woman, who I would later say was my "first angel," told me they could work me in.

After completing the mammogram, I was asked to step into the waiting area. I was called back for an additional procedure, an ultrasound, during which the radiologist came in the room. Dr. B., a petite, young woman, looked at me with caring, compassionate eyes and said, "There are two areas of concern. On the upper, outer right breast there is a two-centimeter, irregular solid mass that looks highly suspicious and an additional cluster of calcifications. You *must* see a surgeon as soon as possible." Her words were deafening and immobilizing. Of course, knowing what I know now and how time is of the essence in matters of health, I believe that the initial technician, who had performed my pelvic ultrasound and arranged for my mammogram to be done that day, was meant to be there. She was meant to work on that day, and at that time, and to be my technician. I was so thankful to her.

An appointment was made with Dr. L., whose demeanor was calm and his smile gentle. He studied the films, examined me, and told me to get dressed so we could talk in his office. Not a good sign, having to "talk" in his office.

He said softly, "Yes, the mass is highly suspicious of a malignancy, and I have spoken with the radiologist. We both agree that the next step is for you to have a stereotactic biopsy." When a mammogram reveals a suspicious area that cannot be felt or is very small, stereotactic core biopsy may be used. I was overwhelmed and couldn't believe what I was hearing. *This can't be happening to me!* Having always been healthy, here I was suddenly and incredulously facing a life-threatening disease. Tears of fear and uncertainty started flowing uncontrollably. I was pinching myself to stop them, but I couldn't. Dr. L. was compassionate, as well as competent, but even he couldn't alleviate my anxiety and sheer terror. I left his office through the back door, still crying, horrified by what was ahead of me. I decided not to tell a soul, except Bert, at least not until I knew the results of the biopsy, which would take an entire week to come back. "Evening and morning, and at noon, will I pray, and cry aloud: and he shall hear my voice" (Psalm 55:17, KJV).

A few days later, I was lying on my stomach on a special table, waiting for the stereotactic core biopsy to begin. My breast was placed through an opening on a mammography table. The biopsy was performed with the guidance of a computer. My breast, pressed between two flat plates (like a mammogram), was X-rayed at various angles. After the suspicious area was identified, the radiologist entered the information into a computer that calculated where the needle would be injected. Dr. B., the radiologist, walked in. I was touched when they asked me, "What kind of music do you prefer?" I really felt like listening to my song of inspiration, "I Will Survive," but I hesitated to ask. Instead, I told Dr. B. that they should choose the music since they were doing all the work and I was just lying there.

The very uncomfortable procedure lasted for about an hour. The nurse's tender touch calmed my fears and was very comforting, while I was told many times to lie completely still and not to move. (It is ironic that, sometime later, I was able to return the support that this nurse provided me. She was diagnosed with breast cancer, and I was there to encourage her and offer hope.) Using a local anesthetic, the instrument moved the biopsy needle into position, and it rapidly removed a sample of the suspicious tissue. It sounded as if they were drilling into my breast. I was so grateful when it was finally over. I drove home with an ice pack placed over the biopsy area inside my bra. The worst part had now arrived: the interminable waiting to find out the results. "Even when I walk through a dark valley, I fear no harm for you are at my side; your rod and staff give me courage" (Psalm 23:4, NAB).

Several anxious days went by without hearing from the doctor's office. I told Bert I wanted to call the doctor but was afraid to hear the results. The following day after I got home from work I did make the call. The office assistant put me on hold to check if the results were back. When she returned on the line she said, "Yes, the results are in, and the doctor will call you when he gets back from surgery."

I pleaded with her, "Please, read what it says. I can't wait any longer. I know it came back positive; if not, you would have said everything is fine."

I felt bad for her because she was only doing her job, and I was putting her on the spot.

She responded very cautiously, "Yes, I am sorry, Mrs. Santamaria, but it is not as bad as you think. It looks like we have caught it at an early stage. The doctor will call you back to explain everything further."

It is horrifying to hear that you have breast cancer. I was frightened, angry, in despair, overwhelmed. I thought, *I am going to die, and I am only forty-six years old!* I thought of my mother-in-law and my father. They had both died from cancer not long after their diagnoses. I also knew that what I was feeling was normal. You go through a grieving period that is very difficult and painful, just as if you have lost a loved one. Eventually, over time, you come to terms with what has happened, and then you start healing.

The phone rang. It was Bert. "Have you heard from the doctor?" I couldn't speak. I could not bring myself to say the words, *I have breast cancer.* There was a pause, complete silence for a while. I couldn't say anything. Then Bert said, "I'll be right home."

When he walked into the house, he looked pale and in disbelief. Only six months had passed since he lost his mother. He was still grieving her death. I knew he was wondering, *Will I lose my wife, too?*

We hugged and I let out a crying scream from deep inside me. The phone rang, and this time it was the doctor. He further explained the results of the biopsy, but wanted to meet with us in his office the next day. That night I could not sleep. All I kept thinking was, *how can I help my family cope with my cancer?* How and when will it be the best time to tell my children and my mother? She was living in Miami at the time. We were born in Cuba. Most elderly

Spanish women will not even say the word *cancer*, out of fear of the disease. How would she react? I was actually afraid she might have a nervous breakdown or a heart attack. Should I wait till I have the surgery? Do I fly her in and tell her in person? Over the phone would be too traumatic. She had gone through a lot taking care of my father when he was diagnosed with cancer. I knew those memories would come back to her. Bert held me in his arms and we prayed until I fell asleep. "I will lie down and sleep in peace, for you alone, O Lord, make me dwell in safety" (Psalm 4:8, NIV).

Bert went with me to the surgeon's office. We were given the last appointment of the day. Dr. G., one of the other surgeons in the practice, spoke to us since Dr. L. was out of town. He was very apologetic because we had been waiting for over an hour to see him (he'd been called in to do an emergency surgery). Dr. G. made us feel very comfortable and was reassuring—I honestly felt he cared about what Bert and I were going through. He explained, "You are in the category that gives you the option to choose between having surgery to remove the entire breast (mastectomy) and underarm lymph nodes, or to remove only the tumor and varying degrees of the remaining breast tissue (lumpectomy)." It is important to note that the option to choose is not available for some types of cancer. He went on. "The treatment recommendation will probably be radiation and chemotherapy with a lumpectomy, and chemotherapy with a mastectomy." He recommended that I make an appointment with a radiation oncologist and a medical oncologist to help me make my choice between a lumpectomy or a mastectomy. The oncologists would determine the best treatment for my type of cancer after they received the pathology report following surgery. The treatments recommended depend on a patient's age, medical history, the type of breast cancer, and how advanced it is. Dr. G. said, "With the mastectomy, you can opt for immediate breast reconstruction or we can delay it for a later time." He suggested I meet with a reconstructive plastic surgeon to find out if I was a candidate for it and to learn more about the procedure. I left the doctor's office determined to put my fears and emotions aside so I could focus on and think very clearly about the crucial decisions concerning my treatment. I needed to be informed. "I will instruct you and teach you in the way you should go; I will guide you with my eye" (Psalm 32:8, NKJV).

The diagnosis of breast cancer is followed by days and weeks of consultation and information gathering. I made an appointment with the plastic surgeon, the oncologist, and the radiation oncologist. The time between the initial diagnosis and the surgery is very stressful. I could not stop asking myself, *am I making the right decision?*

After meeting with the plastic surgeon, I learned that I was a candidate for the free flap TRAM (transverse rectus abdominus myocutaneous) procedure. It can be done by using the woman's own body tissue or with implants. I was in awe that even though I was going to lose such a feminine part of my body, science had made it possible to have a new breast reconstructed.

The time had come to tell my family. I prayed for strength so I would not break down when I told them. "Be strong and courageous. Do not be terrified; do not be discouraged, for the Lord your God will be with you wherever you go" (Joshua 1:9, NIV).

On Valentine's Day, Danny had planned to give his girlfriend, Carolyn, an engagement ring. I did not want to ruin this joyous occasion for them so I waited a couple of days after Valentine's Day to tell him. Danny was very supportive. He said, "Mom, I know you will come out of this an even stronger person. I love you with all my heart." Later, I found out he had hardly slept that night. I now dreaded telling Jaclyn the terrible news that would also put her at a higher risk for developing breast cancer. My voice sounded strong as I spoke. But there was silence on the other end of the line. I reassured her that it looked like we had caught the cancer at an early stage. Jaclyn started to cry. I longed to hug her and comfort her. I thought to myself, *I'm so sorry, my sweet daughter, to hurt you this way.* It is as much of a shock for your family to hear this news as it is for you. But I knew how important it was to keep the lines of communication open, not to shut them out. Your family wants to be a part of your recovery; let them. It makes them feel good to be able to offer their love and support too.

Next, I called my mother. I decided to tell her in person and invited her to visit us. She agreed and I immediately made her flight reservations. I then called my niece, Mariela, who is a registered nurse. When I told her what I was going through, she said, "If you need me, I will get on a plane right now." I knew she meant it.

That weekend, Bert and I drove to Savannah. We wanted to reassure Jaclyn that everything was going to be fine. I also met with Jaclyn's father-in-law, who is a physician, to discuss my options. I left Savannah having made the decision to have a mastectomy with immediate breast reconstruction.

Surgery was set for the last week of February. The day before surgery, I took the Marta train to the airport to pick up my mother. During the ride, she asked me, "Elenita (Spanish people add 'ita' to a name as a form of endearment), is everything okay with you?"

I couldn't keep it from her any longer. "Mom, I am going to say something that is going to sound horrible to you, but really it is not." I spoke confidently and as calmly as possible. I ended by saying, "Cancer is not a death sentence anymore. There are many survivors out there, and I am going to be one of them. I need your love, support, and prayers." Much to my surprise, she handled it very well. She is a very religious and spiritual woman, and I was glad that she was with me. I felt a huge weight had been lifted right after I told her. For the first time in almost a month, I felt pretty good. I was ready for my surgery. "A heart at peace gives life to the body" (Proverb 14:30, NIV).

When I arrived at the pre-op area, I felt I was at a party, and I was the guest of honor. The nurses were waiting for me, making jokes and making me laugh. I was so grateful to them. They helped relieve the tension and anxiety my family and I were feeling. Since I worked on the surgery floor, I had become very close to the nurses. When they heard I had breast cancer, the support and love they expressed was truly what kept me going every day. Other coworkers stopped in to wish me well, including the hospital chaplain. We held hands and prayed just before they wheeled me into surgery. "Your faith has made you well; go in peace, and be healed of your disease" (Mark 5:34, NRSV).

I tolerated the five-hour surgery very well. Bert, Jaclyn, and my mother were in the room waiting for me. Danny had wanted to fly up for the surgery, but I told him not to—he had a new job and I didn't want him to miss work. We would keep him informed. Later, I regretted telling him this, and he said he should not have listened to me.

The nursing care was excellent—my nurse would come in frequently to check the TRAM flap (reconstructive breast) every hour. This is done for a twenty-four-hour period to make sure the circulation and color of the skin is good. Bert went home to get a good night's sleep, and Jaclyn and my mother stayed with me. It was midnight when I awakened to a lot of commotion. Several nurses were at my bedside, surrounding me. I knew something must be terribly wrong. My nurse detected that the TRAM flap was not warm and the color had changed. The plastic surgeon was contacted, and he rushed to my room. He telephoned Bert and said he was going to perform emergency exploratory surgery. My poor husband was paralyzed with fear as he quickly dressed and drove down I-75 at ninety miles an hour to get back to the hospital. Luckily, it was one in the morning—no traffic, no cops.

The plastic surgeon found a small hematoma, a blood clot that forms outside a blood vessel. It is a complication that may arise with this type of surgery, which is why the nurses check the TRAM flap so often.

The first time I got out of bed was quite a challenge. I remember walking very slowly and crookedly down the hospital corridor. My mother and Jaclyn walked on either side of me because I was so weak. And then we laughed—they did not realize it, but in trying to help me, they were walking crookedly down the hallway as much as I was. Every day I showed improvement. The breast health coordinator stopped in to see me. She was indeed another of my "angels." She met with me just after I was diagnosed, and gave me a wealth of information, and introduced me to The Wellness Community. I had gone to my first breast-cancer support group before my surgery and found it to be an invaluable experience. I was able to speak with and ask so many questions of women who had gone through the same type of surgery that I was about to undergo. It was comforting and inspiring to speak to survivors. Now, when the breast health coordinator came to see me, she showed Jaclyn how to do a breast self-examination, and gave me a Susan G. Komen Breast Cancer bear, which was soft and cuddly, with a pink ribbon embroidered on her paw. You hold her under your surgery arm for comfort and support, and squeeze her paw to exercise the arm, which helps maintain good circulation and avoid lymphedema. I left the hospital with my new, cuddly little friend, my new breast, and two out of the four dangling drains. And what a relief it was to receive my pathology report: there had been no lymph node involvement.

With the help of Bert and my mother, I recuperated well from the surgery. It was time for my mom to return to her home in Miami. We had been living in a crowded, tiny, one-bedroom apartment with one bathroom while we house hunted. My mother had been sleeping on an inflatable bed in the living room, surrounded by unpacked boxes, but she never complained. All she wanted was to be there to help with my recovery. She made me the best homemade soups, and every morning we would walk through the beautiful gardens of the apartments. The cliché "take time to smell the roses" really made sense to me now. I was grateful to be alive, but scared of what the future held.

What I dreaded the most, more than my surgery, was chemotherapy. Before my mother left, Jaclyn came up from Savannah to say goodbye to her. We all decided to attend a program entitled Look Good . . . Feel Better. It offers instruction by volunteer cosmetologists on how to apply makeup. They teach women how to draw eyebrows since all body hair is lost to chemo, and give information and suggestions on wigs, turbans, and scarves. They even provide a complimentary makeup kit to each participant. We were surprised when three of the women took off their wigs and were completely bald! (I could not even tell they were wearing wigs.) And all three were laughing and having a good time. They made this very difficult stage seem not quite so horrifying after all. I was so glad that we attended the program because my mother and Jaclyn left feeling better about what I was going to encounter next. So did I.

At the hospital's boutique, A Woman's Place, I bought my first wig. The women who run the boutique are breast-cancer survivors. What should I do with my hair? Their suggestion: cut it short and then shave it. That way you have control. While I was very apprehensive about being there, I found myself having a good time selecting my "new look." I tried many wigs. Jaclyn and my mother would either give me the thumbs up or thumbs down. Finally, one of the women brought out what she called the "hot" wig. It was synthetic, but looked very natural, and it was easy to take care of. It was very short, straight, red with blond highlights—nothing like my own hair. I tried it on and we all knew that was the one! It looked like a fun wig. Plus, it was surprisingly lightweight, which was good since I'd be wearing it through the hot summer. I bought a couple of turbans and a pretty, light blue, soft one to wear to bed. I decided I did not want anyone to see me bald—not even Bert.

In mid-March, I had an appointment with Dr. A., my oncologist.

After my first visit with her, I felt confident that she would be there to make sure I made it through my chemotherapy experience. She explained that I would be having four cycles of Adriamycin and Cytoxan. I did not want to hear this. I was hoping she would say, "No, you don't need chemo after all." She scheduled me for a MUGA (multi-gate acquisition) scan of my heart. We needed to make sure my heart was strong enough because Adriamycin can be quite toxic to the heart. A nurse explained to me the side effects of chemo. I left that appointment with a migraine that lasted for three days. Not only had I just lost a body part, now I was about to lose my hair. I felt I was losing control.

It was time to revisit The Wellness Community. I decided to try visualization techniques and attend the support group. Visualization helps to manage stress, increase energy, and boost the immune system. I hoped it would help get rid of my migraines.

My first chemotherapy infusion was scheduled for the last week of March. Bert wanted to accompany me, but I told him it was best that he go to work. "Just drop me off and don't forget to pick me up," I said. I took with me my prayer books, bottled water, lunch, and a story about surviving breast cancer. As I waited in the lobby, a man in his late fifties came over to me. He must have noticed how scared I looked and that I was alone. Everybody else seemed to have friends or family with them. He sat down next to me and told me the surprising fact that he had advanced-stage breast cancer. I knew men could develop breast cancer, although it's not common. (Approximately 1,400 men are diagnosed each year compared to more than 200,000 women.) He was living each day to the fullest and looking forward to a trip with his grown children. His wife of thirty years had left him after he was diagnosed. He told me that humor had helped to keep him going—it has a healing effect. As he shared his story with me, I felt so sorry for him. How devastating for a man to have a disease that is most common in women. I was very touched and impressed by how he was handling everything. He said I was lucky to have been diagnosed at an early stage. My chances of surviving were high. I thought to myself, *how ironic that I'm being inspired by a man with breast cancer*! He talked to me until I was called. I got up and thanked him for sharing his story and for his words of inspiration, and we wished each other the best. At that moment I realized that if I survived this, I wanted to use my experience to help others who are battling this devastating disease. As the nurse started my chemo, I opened my prayer book and began to pray for myself and for the kind man I had just met.

I was extremely tired after the long day in the treatment room, and glad to be back home late that afternoon. The anti-nausea medication was working; in fact, I was apparently tolerating the treatment rather well. A week and a half after the initial chemo treatment, the first thing I would do every morning when I woke up was to look at my pillow to see if my hair had started to fall out. I realized that losing my hair, even though it would grow back, was going to be even more traumatic than losing my breast! After all, I had awakened from surgery with a beautifully reconstructed breast. But soon I would be waking up *every day* with a bald head, a constant reminder of the disease. I was afraid to go out. I did not know what to expect. Would my hair begin to fall out without warning? I did not want to be in public when it occurred. Then it happened. One morning as I was brushing my hair, I noticed my brush was full of hair. I got in the shower and started shampooing. Clumps of hair fell and fell. I cried quietly as I felt my hair slipping over my wet body. I quickly got out of the shower and started drying what was left of my hair—it was now all over the towel. I could see now why I had been told to shave it, but I hadn't been able to bring myself to do it. I wanted to hold on to my hair for as long as I could. One morning, I woke up and looked at myself in the mirror. I was completely bald except for a handful of hair on the right side of my head. I looked horrible and sickly. My scalp was so sensitive that it constantly hurt.

I started crying and screaming, *"I want my old life back! Who are you? Where is Elena?"* I wanted my soul to leave this body that had betrayed me and live in a healthy one.

Food now tasted unpleasant. I had a metallic taste in my mouth and lost my appetite. It took a great effort for me to eat anything. I started drinking Ensure to supplement what little I was eating. I developed chronic fatigue. My bones hurt, I was tired, I wasn't eating, wasn't sleeping. I lost so much weight that my oncologist warned me not to lose any more. I lost interest in life. . . . I fell into a deep depression.

The house that we had just moved into, and that I had fallen in love with at first sight, I now despised. It had no fond, happy memories. No memories of my children growing up in it, no memories of friends or family gatherings—only memories of my cancer. It did not feel like my home, but a "cancer house."

When I awoke in the mornings, just getting out of bed was difficult. My first thoughts were fears and doubts. Will I ever be happy again? Will I be able to laugh again? Will I have the strength to prepare a Thanksgiving dinner for my family? Will I live to see my grandchildren? Every morning I would go downstairs to the basement where we had built a "mother-in-law suite" for my mother—she had moved from Miami two months after I began my chemotherapy. I would give her a hug and start crying. Then I would ask her to pray with me. As the day progressed, I would start to feel better. But at night it was very hard for me to sleep. I would be awake for hours, even though the doctor had prescribed sleeping pills. The sad routine would start again the following day. I felt I was falling into a deep, dark hole. I tried to climb out, but I couldn't. I remember driving alone in my car, and in the midst of intense grief, I would let out these deep screams within my heart to help relieve the emotional pain. I was desperate and realized I couldn't go on living like this. If I was an emotional and psychological wreck, it would soon impact my immune system. I decided to call the breast health coordinator at the hospital who had helped me so much when I was first diagnosed. She suggested I seek professional help and recommended someone through the hospital's employee assistance program. I saw a counselor for four sessions, was diagnosed as clinically depressed and referred to a psychiatrist. The psychiatrist put me on an antidepressant. Now, I was more worried about my depression than my cancer! She then referred me to a psychologist, who treated me for another year. I poured out all of my hurt, fears, and struggles during our therapy sessions.

Thank God for family and friends through this dark period. The "light at the end of the tunnel" is much farther away without their love and support. I also had a cousin who, a few years before, had been diagnosed with breast cancer. She underwent a lumpectomy, then radiation therapy. We now spoke often on the phone. And I had a dear friend in Florida who had a mastectomy—she was a great source of information and support as well. Another cousin, Carolina, who is a very spiritual person, took a strong interest in my recovery. One day she called to tell me that she had visited an elderly friend of hers. As she was leaving, the old woman said, "I have a gift for you. Here, I want you to have this angel." It was an angel figurine with beautiful, long, golden hair and a very peaceful, lovely face. The angel was praying in a kneeling position. It was a thoughtful gift, my cousin recalled, but upon arriving home, she had a strong sense that this angel was not actually intended for her. A couple of weeks later, she received the news that I had been diagnosed with breast cancer. She knew then that the angel was meant for me. She said to me, "This angel is praying for you. I know you are going to survive all of this. And I know that once you have completed your treatment, once you feel healthy again, you will happen upon another angel. Only this time, the angel will be in an upright, standing position, a sign of your complete healing and recovery." These were truly meaningful words to me and so very needed. When I received the angel, I carefully put it in a special place in my bedroom, right next to my bed.

Later, once I had completed my treatment and was feeling quite good, I drove to Miami with my mother to visit Carolina. When I stopped for gas, I noticed that the gas station had a small store. I decided to go in, taking advantage of the opportunity to stretch my legs. Inside the store, as I was looking at various sundries, I suddenly stopped in my tracks. Of all places to find such a precious thing. I called my mother to show her what I had stumbled upon.

"That's the angel, isn't it?" she asked calmly.

"Yes," I replied. "She is standing, just like I had expected, and of all times to find her, when I am on my way to see Carolina!"

*   *   *   *   *

One thing I learned is that it is very therapeutic to laugh, especially about our cancer experiences. After my chemo was finished, as a reward to my body for all it had endured, I went for my first-ever body massage. Anita, the massage therapist, was a petite, funny, young woman.

Prior to getting started she asked, "Would you like me to massage your scalp?"

"Oh no, thank you," I said. "I'm wearing a wig and don't want to take it off."

She started massaging my back. When she asked me to flip over, somehow, as I turned, my wig fell off. There was silence for a moment. There I was, completely bald. No one had seen me like that except Bert, until now. I burst out laughing.

Anita said, "Well, I guess I'll do your scalp now." And you know what? It felt great!

One event that helped me surface from my depression was the Avon Breast Cancer 3-Day Walk. More than 3,000 walked sixty miles in three days, raising money for a cure. How empowering! Here were strangers sacrificing their free time to train for the long walk. Young women who could be having fun with friends, mothers who could be spending time with their children, retirees who could be out golfing or playing tennis. Instead, they chose to help others. It was inspirational to me. I said to myself: *Snap out of this depressive state. Join them. Do something positive instead of dwelling on the negative. There are people I have never even met fighting for me. Don't give up; join them.*

I wanted to walk with them, but had just finished my chemotherapy and still felt pretty weak. I decided that I would walk the following year, but would participate this year as a crew member. I convinced Bert to join me—it was time to give back what we had received. We signed up for the lunch crew. The first walker I handed a lunch to was a young man. He had one of those big, round picture-buttons on his T-shirt. I said, "What a beautiful lady."

He replied, "That was my wife. I'm walking in her honor. She died last year of breast cancer—she was only forty-three years old." I felt so sorry for him, but also proud of him for honoring her in this way.

For three days we worked very hard, but every minute was worth it. We served lunch to all the walkers and cheered them on. I found myself shouting old Spanish cheers. Many of the walkers would repeat them after me. I was having fun, laughing and crying with everyone, many of whom were survivors. I told my family I was definitely walking next year. They said I would never make it. I was determined to prove them wrong, and, more important, I needed to prove to myself that I was back . . . healthy and full of energy. I had survived chemo; nothing could stop me now.

One year later, a headline in the *Atlanta Journal-Constitution* read: "$5 MILLION, THREE DAYS, ONE CAUSE: BEAT BREAST CANCER." Bert and I, along with 3,000 other walkers, proudly participated in Avon's memorable, powerful event. On our T-shirts, we inscribed the names of loved ones submitted by many of the donors. We dedicated each mile of the walk to them—sixty miles in three days—to honor women and men who have survived breast cancer, those who continue to fight, and those whose battle was lost. Between Bert and me, we raised more than $5,000.

Just five months prior, Bert and I had started our training. On the weekends we would wake up around five o'clock and start walking before sunrise. Our goal was to increase the number of miles each week until we were able to do twenty miles in one day. Then we would do a couple of back-to-back twenty-mile walks before the event. We joined several walking groups from different parts of the greater-Atlanta area to train with them. One day early in our training, we decided to walk at Kennesaw Mountain, north of Atlanta. We started hiking up the mountain. On our way back, we mistakenly took the wrong trail. It wasn't long before we realized that we were lost. Completely lost. To make matters worse, we were running out of water and snacks, and the afternoon was very hot. We couldn't find anyone for help. A little panic and a lot of exhaustion were setting in, but we kept on going. Finally, we heard some distant voices that seemed, we hoped, to be getting closer. We were quite relieved when those voices materialized into two men with their dogs. They said we were pretty close to the visitor's information building at Kennesaw Mountain and told us how to get there. By the time we got to the visitor's center, we realized that we had walked steadily for more than four hours. We both decided the Avon walk would be a piece of cake now.

The first day of the walk, we were completely drenched by a constant deluge of rain. On the last day of the event, my knee was in a lot of pain. Just a month before the walk, a van had rear-ended my car. Not only was my car completely totaled, but I noticed that when I overexerted myself, the pain in my knee would intensify. I had trained for too long and too hard to cancel the walk. So, although the event got off to a painful start for me, it culminated on a beautiful sunny Sunday afternoon with the sounds of loud cheers and nonstop applause at Piedmont Park in downtown Atlanta. The physical therapist had wrapped my knee very tightly to keep it from hurting, but it caused an incredible burning sensation where the tape met my skin. I was almost there, at the finish line; I couldn't quit now. There were people along the route cheering us on, which kept me going. As I approached the finish line, my exhaustion turned into exhilaration. I felt so alive and thankful as the afternoon breeze caressed my face. I had proven to myself that I was healthy and strong again. I could pick up my life where I had left off. As I waved my pink, silk flag that one of the walkers had made for me, I triumphantly crossed the finish line. I was frantically looking for our daughter, Jaclyn, when I heard a high-pitched scream, "Mooommm!" Jaclyn was running toward us, holding our new three-month-old grandson, C. J. My mother was behind her, frantically trying to keep up. I reached out for my mom and my daughter with both arms. Tears of joy and triumph flowed down our cheeks.

* * * * *

The week of Thanksgiving was an extremely busy one that quickly turned into a horrifying scare for me. On Monday, I was scheduled for a routine checkup with my surgeon. On Wednesday, my children and their families would be arriving. Thursday, I had planned a huge Thanksgiving feast. And Friday was Bert's fiftieth birthday. I had invited forty people for a "paella dinner party." On that Monday, as Dr. L. performed my breast exam, he felt a lump in my left breast. An ultrasound was scheduled for the following day.

All the fears and anxiety that I had experienced before now flooded back. Once again, I couldn't believe what I was hearing. I thought, *my cancer is back, and so soon after those grueling months of chemo! I can't believe the chemo did not work.*

I was glad to see Dr. B. walk into the ultrasound room. She was the physician who found the malignant tumor on my mammogram the previous February. She tried to calm my fears.

"Elena, it is probably a liquid-filled cyst that I will aspirate and it will disappear." As she placed the needle in my breast, I noticed that nothing was happening. It was not a liquid-filled cyst but a solid mass. Dr. B. said, "We need to perform a biopsy. Would you like to reschedule for another day or return in the afternoon?"

I replied, "The sooner the better. I'll be back this afternoon." I hurried to my office to tell my boss what was going on. She was very concerned, as was the rest of the staff in the department. Then, I telephoned Bert.

That afternoon the biopsy was performed. It is the time spent waiting for the results that is the most difficult to bear.

I was concerned that if I did not get the results by the following day, Wednesday, I would have to wait until after Thanksgiving. What am I going to do if the results come back positive? And if I have to wait until after Thanksgiving for the results, will I be able to play the part of cheerful hostess without giving away the anguish I'm feeling?

On Wednesday morning when I arrived at my office, I was overwhelmed by what I saw. My desk and the floor around it were covered with red rose petals. There was a gift and a card on my desk from my boss. How very thoughtful and sweet of her to do that. It helped me prepare for what was ahead on this nerve-racking day of waiting for the results.

The day progressed with no word from my physician. I started to get very anxious. As I tried to go about my job, I ran into a female chaplain in the hallway, who was a breast-cancer survivor of nine years. I asked her if she had the time to pray with me in the hospital's chapel. She held my hands and prayed for me as I cried uncontrollably.

"Don't cross the bridge until you come to it," she said. "Have faith in God." I composed myself and left the chapel knowing that no matter the outcome I was going to face it again as an even stronger person.

I received the desperately awaited call late that afternoon. Only this time, it was good news: the tumor was benign. Yes, as a cancer survivor there are days when the thought of a recurrence is terrifying. But it cannot become consuming. Instead, all one's strength should be directed toward healing and coping.

That year, I had the best Thanksgiving of my entire life. There was so much to be thankful for. On Friday, for Bert's fiftieth birthday, I was proud to unveil for him a picture collage that I had been working on for a while. It had photos of all the important events in his life since we met: our wedding, the birth of our children, Bert fishing in his boat, Jaclyn's and Danny's graduation from the university, both of their weddings, and a picture of our family at the beach with our newest family member, our precious grandson, C. J.

I no longer feel that I live in the "cancer house." Instead, it is now a home full of fond memories of a stronger, more united family, of a new me, as I embrace life after breast cancer.

Over the next two years, I would participate in local TV, radio, and newspaper events designed to raise awareness about the importance of early breast-cancer detection. I go out into the community and also reach out to Latino women, speaking about my experience. I teach them the correct way to do breast self-exams. And I've walked in the American Cancer Society Relay for Life and the Susan G. Komen Race for the Cure. My latest challenge was to participate in an Atlanta Falcon's half-time show along with 400 jazzercisers. It was a fundraiser for the Susan G. Komen Foundation. I will keep walking and continue to be a breast-cancer advocate until a cure is found.

❧

A changed woman since her breast cancer, Elena's marriage was challenged in ways that she could not have foreseen. As a result, she and her husband are currently divorcing. At the hospital where she works, she's been promoted from Lead Patient Advocate to Supervisor of Patient Relations. To date, Elena is cancer-free.

Lorna Goldstein

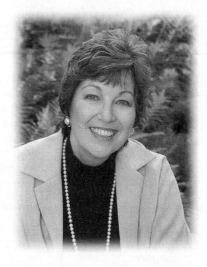

was born and raised in Montreal, Canada. In college, she earned a teacher's certificate with honors in addition to her bachelor's degree. Twenty-two years later, she returned to college to earn a commercial photography certificate. Lorna has traveled the world, accompanying her husband on dozens of business trips. Besides her love for travel and photography, Lorna also likes to paint, as well as play bridge and mah-jongg with her friends. She and her husband, who have been happily married for forty-two years, have two sons and three grand-children. Lorna and her husband reside part of the year at their beloved lake home north of Montreal, and at their Boca Raton house in Florida the rest of the year.

DIAGNOSIS PROFILE

Age at first diagnosis:	45 years old
Family history:	None
Symptoms:	None—abnormal mammogram
Surgery:	Partial mastectomy
	Axillary node dissection
Biopsy results:	Infiltrating ductal carcinoma
	Lymphatic and nerve involvement
	Stage: 1
	Nodes: negative
	Grades: 2 & 3
	Estrogen receptor positive
Radiation therapy:	25 treatments
Age at recurrence:	57 years old
Symptoms:	Swelling, pain in arm and hand, tingling and numbness in fingers. Tumor inoperable due to location

continued on next page

Biopsy results: Metastasis to brachial plexus
Tumor meshed around nerves and artery
Stage: 4
Nodes: none removed
Grade: 2
Estrogen and progesterone receptors positive

Chemotherapy: Taxol
Radiation therapy: 30 treatments
Hormonal therapy: Tamoxifen
Complications: Lymphedema

Additional cancer:
Age at diagnosis: 57 years old
Symptoms: Cramping, spotting, and clotting
Surgery: Total hysterectomy
Biopsy results: Uterine mullerian adenosarcoma
Therapy: No further treatment

I am not dying of cancer. I am living with cancer.

—Unknown

Have Cancer, Will Travel

LORNA GOLDSTEIN

In 1987, when I was forty-five years old, the following conversation took place in a radiologist's office.

"Your mammogram shows calcification. Who is your surgeon?"

"My who? My what? What do you mean?"

"This has to come out, and the sooner the better."

He gave me an envelope with the films and recommended three fine surgeons.

So began my ride on the roller coaster.

*   *   *   *   *

Six months earlier, during a routine annual physical examination, our family practitioner, Dr. S. H., warned of an increased incidence of breast cancer among young Jewish women in the Northeast. We lived in Montreal. This increase in the number of cases apparently was noticed in Montreal, as well as other major eastern cities. He assured me that I was in good health and had no reason for concern; however, he encouraged me to be prudent and not to let more than three years lapse between mammograms. I assured him that I would follow his advice and request a mammogram at my next gynecology examination, which was scheduled in six months.

It was on a Wednesday in late July when I went to see the gynecologist. After the usual examination, he said everything was fine and that he would see me next year. I questioned the need for a mammogram, and with a shrug he said, "If you want one, sure, go get it. I don't feel anything."

He gave me the required requisition, and I immediately went to the radiology center next door, had the mammogram and left.

As I entered my home a short while later, the phone was ringing. I grabbed it just in time to be told by someone at the radiology center that I needed to return for "additional images." My initial reaction was anger, that they had made an error, and that I was being inconvenienced. But on the drive back, it suddenly occurred to me why I had gotten the mammogram in the first place. I was now concerned.

The doctor of radiology personally directed a multitude of angles and magnifications of my right breast. By this time I was growing quite anxious, but was assured I would have the results before I left the center. The doctor finally called me into his office where my films were spread on the viewing boxes. He explained as he marked the problem. "It was almost off the film but was picked up with a magnifying glass. That is why I had you come back. I'm sorry, but . . ."

I don't remember how I managed to drive home that afternoon. After twenty-six years of marriage and raising two sons, I could not recall anything more sobering than this instant reality check: facing my own mortality. I was frightened. My stomach was in knots. My mouth was dry. My mind was working overtime. I vacillated between sobbing and trying to organize my thoughts. By the time my husband,

George, arrived home I feared the worst. Fortunately, we were able to meet with Dr. M., a surgeon, that very evening. After examining me and checking the films, he offered his opinion: because of the pronounced veins and dimpling flesh, he was 90 percent sure it was cancer. "I could be wrong, of course," he said, but recommended I check into the hospital the following Monday for surgery.

I remember being overwhelmed by Dr. M.'s opinion. He had confirmed my worst fears. All this happened within a few hours, but I instinctively knew I would need a second opinion before I could agree to surgery. A few phone calls later, I was given an appointment for the following morning with Dr. R., a renowned breast-cancer specialist. He agreed that surgery could be indicated and suggested a two-step investigation. The first step would be a needle biopsy and then, if necessary, surgery would take place the following week.

How was I going to get through a week of not knowing? What should I do? Which surgeon to use? Dr. M. had a great reputation and was gentle and empathetic. Dr. R. was known for his research work in breast cancer, but I was so intimidated by his manner—cold and businesslike—that I wasn't able to ask even the necessary questions.

It was Friday. Two days had passed since the mammogram. I found it impossible to sleep and was nauseated at mealtime. And since the summer days were upon us, we had family visiting, and a full weekend planned. How could I pretend everything was normal? How could I get through the weekend? How could I decide what to do and which surgeon to use? Resources for gathering information were not readily available. Time was short. George was also in a state of fear and disbelief. He had no insight, no information that would help with the decision.

No one in my family had ever had breast cancer. My parents were healthy. My younger brothers were healthy. No member of my husband's family had been diagnosed with cancer. None of my friends or business acquaintances had cancer. Who could I talk to? Who could help me? My family was there, but I felt alone. There wasn't a soul who could advise me what to do. It would be the first of many decisions that I would make on my own.

I remember that Sunday evening, after dinner, telling our family we had something serious to discuss. I tried to be matter of fact as I told them exactly what had transpired a few days earlier, and that I planned to go into the hospital the next morning. I added, "I need all my energy to fight this disease and I will need your support. If you want to cry, do it privately. Not near me."

Not knowing the facts was worse than facing the truth. I went into the hospital within five days of discovery. It was suggested that I would probably have a segmental section with axillary node dissection; however, the consent form left the decision up to the surgeon should I need a radical mastectomy.

I remember few details of the actual eight-day stay in the hospital. The surgery was a partial mastectomy, a wedge of breast tissue had been removed. I awoke from surgery to terrible news. I was told that the tumor was malignant; some lymph nodes had appeared red and swollen and had been removed. The doctor said I would have to await the pathology to get a final prognosis and treatment. I went into a state of shock. Visitors came and did not know what to say. Many friends stayed away because they also did not know what to say.

The Jewish General Hospital in Montreal is a teaching hospital, and as such, students and medical personnel routinely interviewed me. Some of the questions were personal regarding family medical histories, smoking and drinking habits, and particularly birth control methods, pregnancies, and childbirth. I had never smoked, drank wine occasionally, and had only taken birth control pills for about six months many years earlier. Some questions seemed routine, but others hit a raw nerve. "How old are your children? Are they able to get along without you if necessary?"

Was I going to die from this? Had I suddenly become just a statistic?

Other people came and went: a social worker, a psychologist, and a representative from Hope and Cope, an organization within the hospital that helps both cancer patients and their families. They each introduced themselves, told me of various services available, and encouraged me to call should I need their help.

Immediately after surgery, I was able to deal with the physical issues. But not the emotional. A drain had been inserted into each of the two incisions to remove excess fluids from the surgical sites. The drains, the pain and tenderness, and limited arm movements would eventually disappear. Eight days later, the drains were no longer necessary and were removed. I was sent home with an exercise program to help regain full mobility of my arm and shoulder area.

After several weeks, as soon as I began to feel better physically, I was ready to reach out for other forms of help. It took a lot of energy and determination, but I started with a visit to the support group Hope and Cope. The social worker there suggested I be teamed up with a breast-cancer survivor. She also gave me some books about the disease.

Rebecca was the first person I met who had experienced breast cancer. She was a ten-year survivor (and still cancer-free today) and was able to answer my many questions, as well as help me with some personal issues.

Ibby was another woman who reached out to me. She was a registered nurse involved in a program called NUCARE (Nursing Cancer Rehabilitation and Research), a support program of nurses who work individually with patients. They teach coping skills to assist survivors in regaining control of their lives. We had a one-on-one session of relaxation therapy. I was given a tape and encouraged to take quiet time every day to focus on mind-body relaxation.

Reading about breast cancer became a priority for me. I sought not only to learn more about the disease, but also the encouragement of survivors' stories. Dr. Bernie Siegel became my inspiration. I was also fortunate to attend one of his workshops. From that point on, life became more precious. I no longer wanted to listen to trivialities. I had no patience for nonsense, gossip, or people who constantly complained. I wanted only positive energy and uplifting people around me. I also needed a normal daily existence with my family.

As I was coming to grips with my cancer, those close to me reacted in different ways. All my life I had been a giver, a protector, and a nurturer. Now I needed the energy for myself, and I could not concern myself with other people's fears and problems.

George, my love and greatest supporter for twenty-six years, buried himself in new challenges at work. It took him about six weeks before he could share his feelings and not worry about touching me or upsetting me.

Our sons, Warren and Jeff, for my benefit, appeared to keep life on an even keel. But I was aware of their concerns and frequent glances when they felt helpless to do anything.

My parents, who had always considered me independent and self-sufficient, now offered me a tremendous amount of moral support. It was needed and greatly appreciated.

Several friends told me they were amazed at how "matter of fact" and strong I was. What did they expect? Diane, a very close friend, wanted to take me to a sidewalk café and get drunk. Herby, another friend, called frequently and dropped by sporadically. His approach was, "If you want to talk, cry, or be quiet, I'm here for you." I truly appreciated his visits and phone calls.

"You will need radiation therapy," Dr. M., the breast surgeon, said. My parents drove me to my first appointment, where my chest and neck would be measured and marked. Walking into the waiting room shocked us all. I don't know what I expected but what I saw was depressing. There were patients, young and old, some in wheel-chairs, some with no hair, others in hospital gowns, and several healthy-looking women in street clothes, obviously volunteers. Many were chatting cheerfully, reading magazines, or eating refreshments. *I do not belong here with all these sick people* was what kept going through my mind.

After a Polaroid photo of me was taken and my file opened, I realized that this radiation department would be my center of focus for the next six weeks. *I had better get used to being here*, I thought. Many of the women in street clothes were, in fact, outpatients just like me. In time, it became somehow reassuring to follow the daily routine of treatment. I was doing something to help myself—I was *killing* the cancer cells.

The treatments themselves were painless. They took place in a room similar to the usual X-ray set-up. I reclined on a table with my arm placed horizontally in a *V*-position and my hand rested on my hip. A plastic-looking cone was positioned toward my right breast, and I was instructed to stay very still. The procedure took just a few minutes.

Because the effects of radiation are cumulative, sometimes fair-skinned patients have skin problems by the last week of treatment. After just three days, my breast became swollen and red, as if I had a bad sunburn. Dr. G., the radiation oncologist, expressed concern that my very sensitive skin could possibly compromise my therapy. Fortunately, the irritation did not develop into an infection, and I was able to complete all twenty-five treatments.

During the period of radiation therapy I had specific restrictions: no showers, no soap on the breast, and no deodorant on the right side. I recall the dish of cornstarch and vitamin E oil as part of my daily bathing routine. For several months I could neither wear a bra nor tolerate any tight-fitting clothes.

Then came another extremely difficult decision: whether or not to participate in the protocol offered at that time. I was again referred to Dr. R., who headed the scientific study. Tamoxifen had been successful in treating postmenopausal women, but this new blind study would be on premenopausal women. If I were given the drug, it would bring on early menopause. If I were given a placebo, it would do nothing. Which choice was right for me? Making this decision caused sleepless nights and much anxiety. Family and friends were not knowledgeable, of course, so I could have no confidence in their opinions. I consulted several medical professionals only to receive mixed opinions. One doctor said, "Why use an elephant gun to kill an ant?" Another said that anything Dr. R. recommended was what he would suggest. Back to square one: me.

The final decision had to be mine alone. Dr. R. tried to convince me to participate because the study needed more volunteers. When I asked if he would give me tamoxifen without the study, he refused. I chose not to participate. Now, retrospectively, I sometimes wonder if it was the right decision.

*   *   *   *   *

Twelve years later, at age fifty-seven, I realized I was not sure when my recent symptoms had started. Six years earlier, we had relocated from Montreal to Atlanta, Georgia. It was not a desired move, but George had taken on additional business responsibilities that necessitated the relocation. Up until that time, Montreal had been home for my entire life.

There were many reasons for my not wanting to move to Atlanta. George was a senior executive with a Montreal-based company. His career required worldwide travel to visit with suppliers and customers, and attend trade shows. Once our sons were grown and independent, I was happily able to join George on his business trips. While he was occupied with work during the day, I took the opportunity to go exploring with my camera. I had recently completed several years of study and was now a commercial photographer whose real love was travel photography. In foreign countries, I would frequently go off on my own; however, there were times when I had a guide and driver to escort me. Each exciting adventurous day would end with George and me having dinner, often with his business associates. We usually added a few extra days to each trip for "together" time.

One trip was to Atlanta, where a trade show was in progress. I so looked forward to exploring this southern city—its people, sights, and architecture. Early on our first morning, George set out for the convention center and I took my camera bag, ready for some serious exploring and photographing. As I was going out the door of our beautiful downtown hotel, I was stopped by the doorman, who questioned where I was headed. He was horrified when I told him of my intention to photograph the area. His words still echo in my mind: "You cannot go out there alone. You will be mugged—it's much too dangerous. If you want to go anywhere, take a taxi and go shopping at Lenox Mall."

I was stunned. I had traveled on the train alone in Tokyo. I had explored many neighborhoods in European cities. Here I was, in a lovely American city, being told it wasn't *safe*. Shopping, indeed! I was so angry that I went back up to my hotel room, called room service and ordered lunch, and watched pay-per-view movies all day. When George returned at dinnertime, I was adamant that I never wanted to go to Atlanta again.

My reaction to relocating was also rooted in deeper issues that I thought had long ago been resolved. When I was fourteen years old, my parents left Montreal to start a business in northern Quebec, about 500 miles away. The move was to a remote wilderness region—barely accessible. But my parents were pioneers and looked forward to their adventure. They decided, however, it was in my best

interest to stay in Montreal with relatives and continue my education at a proper high school—as there was only a three-room school-
house where they were relocating. My two brothers, on the other
hand, were younger, and my parents thought that their five-year plan
to live in a mining town would not create a problem for the boys.
And so, the family was splintered, me living in the city, visiting them
only during school breaks, and the four of them living in primitive
conditions behind the store they had opened. It was a situation that
would have a haunting effect on me for many years. The first year or
so was terribly unsettling. I felt abandoned. I moved from one home
to another until finally I found myself in a family environment with
an aunt, uncle, and two cousins. I lived with them for several years,
until a short time before George and I were married.

Thus, my reaction to the news of moving to Atlanta was deeply
emotional, and I truly believed I could not go along with the decision, although our eldest son, Warren, in his wisdom, figured out
why I was so upset. He believed that my abandonment issues were
resurfacing. Only this time, I was doing what I vowed I would never
do: leave my children. Warren reasoned, "Mom, this is different.
We are independent adults. Jeff is married, and I am on my own.
You were only a child. This is not abandonment. If we had an
opportunity to further our careers, we would move too." Bless you,
Son. Today, both boys are married and no longer living in Montreal.

But there was no way I would completely sever my roots to
Montreal and our life there. I insisted on spending six weeks every
summer at our lake house, an hour's drive from the city. With this
concession I agreed to the move, although I was neither excited nor
pleased about it.

Included in my concerns was my medical history with breast
cancer, and because of that, after the move, I decided to maintain
contact with my trusted cancer physicians, Dr. G. and Dr. M., and
had appointments with them on a fairly regular basis. The Montreal

doctors kept reassuring me that the cancer was gone, that I could forget about it. I was frequently reminded to protect my right arm from potential problems of lymphedema, not to use that arm for blood tests and blood pressure cuffs, watch for infection, not to lift heavy objects, etc., and to never take estrogen because my tumor had been estrogen positive. In addition to the medical attention in Montreal, I was also seen yearly in Atlanta by a gynecologist, internist, and breast surgeon. Blood tests and mammograms were done on a regular basis.

Menopause, with all its uncomfortable side effects, particularly hot flashes and night sweats, assaulted me. My Atlanta doctors encouraged me to take estrogen to relieve my menopausal symptoms, as well as to help prevent osteoporosis. I was horrified when the breast surgeon also suggested hormone therapy. My tumor was estrogen positive, which meant that my cancer cells used estrogen to thrive and grow. I asked why she recommended HRT for me, after all these years of being told not to even consider taking estrogen. Her response was, "This is a new era. Things are different. The data is inconclusive regarding the connection of estrogen and the risk of breast cancer. Why should you be miserable with menopause?" That's when I decided to change physicians. Fortunately, I did not go on HRT.

Over the years, I had occasionally complained of a sore neck, arm and/or shoulder, especially after playing golf. When a problem arose, I would consult Dr. J., an orthopedic surgeon and personal friend, who arranged for X-rays, and treated me for rotator cuff injuries, tennis elbow, and similar problems. Treatment was usually physical therapy, anti-inflammatory drugs, muscle relaxants, and/or cortisone injections. This routine occurred every few years, but I always recovered, and my doctors, including the cancer specialists, continued to say, "Don't worry."

Our lives changed when George retired. We sold our home in

Atlanta, relocated to Florida, and embarked on a trip around the world. We flew to London, England, where after three days, the news of a death in the family brought us back to Canada.

We were able to resume our trip and went directly to India, where we spent about a month visiting this fascinating, diverse, spiritual country. In cities, towns, and villages, we were constantly amazed by and enchanted with the diversity of the people, the culture, the street markets brimming with foods and flowers, animals, the pungent mix of people and animal "aromas," the magnificent maharajahs' palaces (some now hotels), mud and dung huts where the women and girls collected water from the village well, the temples, the religious customs, shepherds leading their camels to market, the Taj Mahal, the Red Fort—all contributed to a fabulous photographic experience: ancient times meet the modern world.

Of all the memorable experiences of our trip, one stands out as particularly moving. It was a pre-dawn visit to Varanasi, the holy city on the Ganges River. George and I were in one of the many small boats floating close to shore from where we could witness funeral pyres on the bank and people standing in the water, some bathing, some praying, some doing both. We were each given our own floating candle to light and set afloat with our personal prayers. It was an incredibly spiritual experience to see hundreds of twinkling flames on the water as dawn broke.

After India, we had planned an extended stay in Australia and New Zealand, but on our third day in Sydney, we were once again notified of another death in our family. "Let's just go home and stay home," I said to George. He agreed immediately.

* * * * *

Soon after returning to Florida, I injured my back playing golf. I was undergoing treatment for back pain when I complicated my recovery by tripping over a tree root, landing on pavement and injuring my right hand. Despite this klutzy incident, I managed to finish up the physical therapy for my back, but I was left with numbness in my thumb from the fall. George and I were in our nomadic lifestyle mode, traveling again, and I tried not to let my back and hand problems interfere too much. But over a period of several months, I gradually developed more pain in my upper and lower back, shoulder, neck, arm, and a tingling sensation started in my fingers. Painkillers kept the situation bearable as we continued to travel, but I knew that sooner rather than later, I would have to deal with whatever was going on in my body.

August found us back in Montreal, and I went to see Dr. G., the radiation oncologist who had been following my progress since the breast surgery. When he saw that my arm was swollen and painful to move, he was quick with an opinion. He said it was lymphedema and suggested that I wear a compression sleeve to ease the problem. He reminded me not to carry luggage, not to hold my grandchild, and again, that I must protect my arm. Although it seemed possible that I may have overused my arm, I could not understand why I would develop such a serious problem after having been so careful over the years.

We bought a vacation home in Atlanta in late summer, and while spending time there a few weeks later, I knew I needed additional medical help. I was living with constant and escalating pain. After two weeks and no relief from the usual treatment, Dr. J., the orthopedic surgeon, ordered an MRI of my neck. The results were not impressive and although bone spurs were visible, in his opinion, these spurs should not be causing the extreme pain and tingling in my arm and hand. He referred me to Dr. P., a neurosurgeon.

Dr. P. said that, in light of my history with breast cancer, before he started to explore my spine, he wanted an MRI of the brachial plexus (area between the neck and underarm) on my right side.

There were several days of intense anxiety as I waited for his phone call. Then it came.

"I'm sorry," Dr. P. said. "This is not my field of expertise. Who is your medical oncologist?"

"My who? My what? I don't have one. I never needed one."

> *I'm up. I'm down*
> *I scream and cry*
> *My eyes are wet,*
> *My mouth is dry.*
> *Why me? Why now?*
> *How can this be?*
> *So much to live for*
> *What's happening to me?*

Roller coaster, here we go again! My throat and stomach met. The shock and fears came flooding back. Where to start? Who to use? Do I return to Montreal? Do I need a major cancer center? Should I go to Florida? Should I stay in Atlanta near my family? What should I do? We asked the advice of several Atlanta medical friends, and all referred me to Dr. D., a medical oncologist in Atlanta.

George and I were numb and awkward at the first appointment. We were not prepared. We knew neither what to expect nor the questions to ask. Dr. D. had relocated from South Africa to the U.S., and at times I had difficulty understanding some of the dialogue. He used visual images with markers and diagrams to explain my new problem—my new malignant tumor—but I am not sure how much I grasped. When looking at the illustrations at a later time, I still did not understand all of them. I remember asking why palliative—why not *cure*? Where am I on the bell curve of survival? Why did he bring up a living will? *Was I going to die?*

Dr. D. explained that surgery was not an option because of the nature of the tumor. It had meshed with the nerves and artery in the brachial plexus. This meant that the tumor was not a singular, definable mass, but had grown over and around the nerves and artery. Thus, trying to operate was extremely risky; surgery could cause crippling, permanent disability, or worse. It was explained that this cancer was very unusual, although not entirely rare.

A biopsy was needed, but because of the dangers involved due to the nature of the tumor, it was difficult to find a safe location. The process was long and tedious, done step by step in conjunction with a continuing CAT scan. At the same time, I requested tissue samples from Montreal from my earlier bout with cancer so that the Atlanta doctor could determine if this was a new primary tumor or a metastasis. As it turned out, the tissue samples were alike, both estrogen positive, and I was told that it was very unusual to have metastasized in this manner.

How could this be? I had been assured for twelve years that I had been cured.

Being right-handed, my daily routine was now severely hampered. I could not lift my arm without pain or hold anything in my hand, not even a fork. I was clumsily trying to eat with my left hand, but having a hard time, and I certainly couldn't write left-handed.

Dr. D. suggested that I begin a program of radiation as quickly as possible to control the pain and loss of function. Radiation was the quickest way to reduce the tumor, he said. When Dr. D. consulted with Dr. L. H., the radiation oncologist who would be directing my treatment, they discovered a problem: where to mark the field because of my prior treatment. Part of the tumor was located in an area that had been previously radiated. Because it was critical to know exactly where and how much radiation could be used, I contacted Dr. G. in Montreal and requested my records. He was shocked when I told him of the metastasis. Not as shocked as I was, I assured him.

In Atlanta, my doctors arranged thirty radiation treatments (five days a week) combined with weekly low doses of Taxol. The chemotherapy would be stopped during the last ten days to allow overlap treatment on the original radiated area.

I worried that my sensitive skin might tolerate the radiation as poorly as it did the last time. But I knew I had no choice. It was sunburn or . . . I didn't even want to consider the alternative.

Dr. L. H. measured and marked my chest, arm, and neck, and placed several permanent pinpoint tattoos to outline the new field of radiation. I wondered why this was not done twelve years earlier. It would have made the doctor's assessment and planning much easier. The treatment would be to my chest, back, shoulder, and neck. It was also explained that the field would overlap to part of my thyroid gland and a bit of my right lung. Scarring of that portion of the lung was likely but tolerable, and if the thyroid gland should become a problem, it could be controlled with medication.

The radiation appointments were arranged for early in the morning, affording me a reasonable daily life. My routine was to lie on a bare table with a specific headrest. A technician adjusted my head and neck position, and my right arm was propped up and supported at a ninety-degree angle. My feet were held together with a strap so that I could not move. I thought of people in mental hospitals who had to be restrained in bed—how horrible. The machine was programmed with a block that outlined only the field to be radiated while protecting those areas not to be exposed. A separate block is designed exclusively for each patient. After the table position was adjusted so that the light from the machine lined up exactly with my tattoos, the two technicians did a verbal check before leaving the room. The machine radiated my chest and then turned automatically to do my back.

Once the routine was established it went smoothly . . . until one day during the December holiday season. My regular technicians were on a different scheduled rotation and new, part-time people took their place. Everything that day was unusual. The set-up was strange: the normally bare table was draped with a sheet, a different support was placed under my head, my arm was not aligned or supported, my feet were not tied, my head was in an uncomfortable position, and the usual verbal double-checks between technicians were not done. During the treatment, I felt a burning sensation in my face and my right eye. I called for help. A nurse checked me over and then a doctor. The right side of my face was red and the area around the eye was swollen. No question: something had gone wrong! I was later told that they may have "tweaked" the sympathetic optic nerve that runs close to the radiated field and up through the face. Although the doctor assured me it was not an error, I believed differently. The next day, I followed up with visits to my radiation oncologist and ophthalmologist; both told me they were sure there would be no lasting effects. I'm happy to say they were right. The rest of the treatments were done very carefully with the proper verbal checks and controls.

For the most part, my skin tolerated the treatments well. The only problem was when a collar touched a portion of my neck where the skin was irritated and moist. I had to wear cotton padding on my neck to act as a buffer and apply an antibiotic ointment to the delicate area. That portion of the radiation field had to be blocked for the last ten days of treatment.

Chemotherapy would be a new experience for me. The protocol ordered was four consecutive weeks of low-dose Taxol in conjunction with the radiation therapy. The simultaneous treatments, hopefully, would attack all areas of tumor that radiation alone could not reach, as well as enhance the radiation field. The unknown has always been difficult for me. The idea of chemotherapy frightened me. I was back on my roller coaster again.

The location for administering the chemotherapy would be in a wing adjacent to Dr. D.'s office, not in the hospital. I was pleasantly surprised to find the place large and bright, not the antiseptic environment I had envisioned. There were numerous recliner chairs arranged in small groups. Each area was equipped with a television, VCR, headsets, audiotapes, and magazines. I found male and female patients of various ages and in all stages of illness. Unlike twelve years ago, I was not frightened by what I saw.

Each chemotherapy treatment was preceded by a blood test and depended on its favorable results. Because of all the scans and tests I had been subjected to over the years, the veins in my left arm were very fragile. The receptionist greeted me with a spongy peach and suggested I squeeze frequently to ease her finding a vein. She also suggested I request the "one-stick procedure," which would allow for both the drawing of blood and the receiving of the intravenous drips. To prepare me for paclitaxel IV (Taxol), I was first infused with dexamethasone (Decadron), diphenhydramine (Benadryl), and cimetidine (Tagamet) to reduce the potential for nausea and allergic reaction, and also to relax me. The Taxol drip followed. This would be the standard procedure for each weekly infusion.

The initial Taxol dose was infused very slowly to be sure I could tolerate it well. A pump regulated the amount and speed of the drugs administered, while a nurse monitored the infusion and made adjustments as the session progressed. One day, the procedure was suddenly interrupted by a flurry of activity around my chair. A mistake had occurred—it was not my bag of Taxol! Fortunately, the error was caught quickly, and although the medication was also Taxol, this bag had been measured for someone else. They had not verified the name on the bag. Of course, mistakes like this should never happen. It was then I realized that everyone and everything had to be checked and rechecked, and that some aspects of treatment are in the patient's hands. This episode was brought to the attention of the doctor and the administration, who assured me they would investigate their monitoring procedures more thoroughly in the future. A small consolation.

With chemotherapy came other challenges. I was given an information package about Taxol and prescriptions to cover the typical side effects: constipation, diarrhea, nausea, anxiety, and sleeplessness. I filled all the prescriptions, but lucky me, I did not need to use them. I expected to have hair loss, and so I shopped around for a wig. I watched daily as my hair thinned out, but in the end, a short, stylish haircut was all I needed.

The combined treatment was working. The pain and numbness in my arm and hand gradually subsided. Within a few weeks, and for the first time in a long time, I needed only a minimal amount of pain medication. But fatigue was a new experience, coming as a byproduct of chemotherapy and radiation, and daily power naps became mandatory.

Dr. D. further recommended both lymphedema treatments and physical therapy to aid in regaining use of my arm and hand. During my investigation of lymphedema programs, I discovered a variety of options. Some treatments required lymphatic drainage and/or bandaging, a three-hour daily commitment for up to six weeks. Another approach was a compression sleeve and pump.

Dr. L. H. referred me to a physical therapist, Robbie, who specialized in therapy for breast-cancer patients. Robbie worked with me twice a week for both the lymphedema and mobility. She regularly measured my arms to assess the progress. With massage, exercises, and layers of cotton bandaging, my condition quickly improved. My visits to Robbie were reduced to once a week, and with her training, I was taught to bandage myself and was given an exercise program to do at home. The swelling was significantly reduced and my mobility improved. I could once again raise my arm over my head. What a feat! Most exciting, though, was regaining the use of my fingers and hand. Little things like holding a fork, cutting my food, and signing my name took on a whole new meaning. How much we take for granted is one of the prime lessons. My strength and flexibility gradually returned. However, I was left with residual tingling in the hand and fingers. The doctor explained that some of the nerves in my arm were compromised for too long a period of time. They would not regenerate. Very fine motor skills, like threading a needle and sewing, required watching my hand and finger movements very closely because I could not feel the needle. Although I regained the agility, my sense of touch was limited. A small price to pay.

Throughout those few months my roller coaster was up and down. The successes were exhilarating highs, but the fears and anxieties were horrible lows. I learned that some of my stress was related to the "unknown," always assuming the worst-case scenario. The realities I was able to deal with, but my fears brought periods of depression. Dr. D. recommended that I learn how to assess the real issues from those imagined. Meditation, yoga, and T'ai Chi came to the rescue. The mind-body relaxation was enjoyable and calmed me to the point that I was finally able to separate the real from the imagined. It was an inexpressible relief.

During this same period, while I was undergoing testing and treatments, George was with me all the time. His positive perspective, inspiration, and encouragement counteracted my depression. His relief at my having successfully gone through these treatments, and my reaction to his optimistic approach, gave us the impetus to resume a more normal life.

I started to attend workshops and meetings at various Wellness centers in Atlanta. Three programs that were the most significant to me were: Coping with Anger, Dream Interpretation, and Stress Management.

I had not realized how angry I was. For several years after my first bout with breast cancer, I was aware of the risks and concerns of recurrence. But after five years, and then ten years, I gradually dropped my guard. Now I became angry with my doctors for encouraging me to forget it and put it behind me. I was angry with my husband, his career, and our nomadic lifestyle. Although it was exciting and glamorous to travel much of the year and have homes in several locations, I missed the stability of staying in one place, and I often wondered if it had caused me to "fall through the cracks," medically speaking. I was conscientious with my annual examinations, as well as mammograms, but was there something I had overlooked?

The biggest surprise was to realize I was mostly angry with myself. How could I have permitted this to happen? Could I have been more aware and acted sooner? Would it have made a difference? It was imperative that I come to terms with this anger and realize I could not change the past. Once I was able to recognize the source of my anger, I was able to get rid of it. Finally, I would focus on the positive aspects of life, even life itself.

For many weeks I had difficulty sleeping. I was restless and tense and my mind worked overtime. Every third or fourth night, I took medication to help me catch up on my much-needed rest. It was suggested in a Wellness program to stop the pills and allow the fears and concerns to surface. I was encouraged to keep a journal and to "go with the feelings" as they emerged. It is amazing how much easier it is to deal with issues when you face them. I was also encouraged to concentrate on positive thoughts and affirmations.

Another form of therapy that helped me tremendously was spending time outdoors. Nature walks became an integral part of my well-being. Trees, water, birds, and flowers soothed my mind and reconnected me with the natural beauty that surrounds us—something we too often take for granted.

Dream interpretation was another healing and revealing workshop experience. I had had a nightmare of a little girl playing outside. I could not see her face, only her back, but her clothes were familiar and I knew exactly where she was. When someone called out to her, she responded to my name. I awakened startled. I am an Ashkenazi Jew, and it is our tradition to name newborns after a deceased relative. I just knew that night I was going to die and that I had seen my namesake, my granddaughter, in my dream.

When discussing my dream with the interpreter, she completely turned it from dying to living. The little girl was familiar. In my childhood album there is a picture of me at the same place, wearing the same clothes. Her interpretation was that the young Lorna wanted to come out and play. She suggested that I enlarge the picture of myself and place it where I could be encouraged to be "young at heart" again.

Once I came to believe that I was not *dying* of cancer, but rather *living* with cancer, I realized the need to research my situation. Along with books, the Internet provided many options. George spent days gathering information on breast cancer, but there was very little about my particular form of metastasis.

We decided to consult with three major cancer centers: Memorial Sloan-Kettering in New York, M. D. Anderson in Houston, Texas, and Dana Farber in Boston. At each facility I was examined by a medical oncologist who reviewed my records, scans, and slides. All agreed that the therapy I had received was the best one for me. When I asked whether there were any clinical studies in which I was eligible to participate, I was told that there might be one in about six months in New York, but that I should carefully weigh the pros and cons before joining. It would require frequent trips, hotel stays, side effects, and just possibly it might not help. At present, I still don't know what I would do should a new clinical trial become available.

Alternative medicine and nutritional changes were other options I explored. How could I help my immune system fight this disease? In this case, I'm afraid I encountered conflicting medical opinions. By and large, the scientific community does not embrace holistic medicine. And I must admit, some of the suggestions were extreme and unconventional. But I was surprised at how little *conclusive* information I was able to glean from doctors. It was, of course, a major frustration for me. Eventually, I settled on a regimen of healthy eating with some vitamin supplements.

With radiation and chemo behind me, I started taking tamoxifen, the same anti-estrogen medication proven years ago to help postmenopausal women. Hot flashes and night sweats were reminders of menopause, but they were a small inconvenience when I looked at the big picture. I was alerted to the risk of other side effects of tamoxifen, but my needs undoubtedly justified the risks.

Medically, for the first year after the metastasis was diagnosed, the doctors monitored me every three months with regular clinical examinations, blood tests, CAT scans checking lungs, abdomen, and pelvis, and MRI of the brachial plexus. Unfortunately, the scans were not able to accurately evaluate my progress—it was impossible to measure just the tumor because the area is a complex mass of tissue, network of nerves, artery, and scar tissue. The doctors have now suggested fewer scans to avoid the risk of over-radiating me. They said my progress would have to be evaluated more with clinical visits, blood tests, and the subjective evaluation of how my fingers, hand, and arm were functioning. I was also advised to be extremely watchful of any new problems or symptoms that lingered more than a few weeks. They would need to be investigated because the cancer could return elsewhere.

And so with this nightmare behind me, George and I left Atlanta and returned to Florida—a welcome reprieve from medical appointments. Being outdoors again in the sunshine and balmy breezes was wonderful. My plans for recuperation included walking daily along the beach, eating healthily, and reading about things *other* than cancer.

* * * * *

A mere two weeks later I was back on my roller coaster. This time with symptoms of cramping, spotting, and clotting. How could this happen four years after menopause? I was not on estrogen. Something must be wrong; these symptoms were not "normal." I hastily returned to Atlanta and saw my gynecologist, Dr. A. She immediately recommended a dilation and curettage (D&C). More blood tests, X-rays, ultrasound, biopsy, and pathology. Diagnosis: a low-grade mullerian adenosarcoma. In other words, another cancer! I would need a hysterectomy at once. Dr. A. recommended that I consult with an oncology gynecologist to perform the operation. Another doctor, another problem.

Dr. D., my quarterback throughout the last several months, concurred with Dr. A. For the moment, it was out of his hands. When I asked if this was the second shoe falling, he told me I was like an octopus with many legs. He also said to look at this as a gift: Now I would no longer have to worry about the risk of uterine cancer from tamoxifen!

I tend to believe that good often comes from something bad. The traditional surgical method for a hysterectomy was an abdominal incision to excise the necessary organs. The recuperation period was lengthy and difficult. A newer and easier method, laparoscopic surgery, involves making four small holes in the navel and pelvic areas, and removing the organs vaginally. I was fortunate to have the vaginal hysterectomy and could look forward to a quick physical recuperation.

Emotionally, I did not bounce back as fast. During a period of six months, I had been diagnosed with metastatic breast cancer, and then (unrelated) uterine cancer. Too much bad news, coming at me too fast. With all the testing, biopsies, diagnoses, treatments, pain, medication, surgeries, anxieties, not to mention hospital stays and doctor visits, my emotional roller coaster was ready to jump off the track. Just as I was getting stronger, physically and emotionally— *bam!*—another scary setback hit me.

For almost four decades, George and I had been involved in philanthropic causes. Our focus now became breast-cancer support and research. October is breast-cancer awareness month, and there are many opportunities nationwide to show support, actively and financially. In Atlanta, we had our chance to participate in the Susan G. Komen's "Race for the Cure." This annual event is open to survivors and supporters. The day's program consists of registration, then the actual walk or run, followed by a festive gathering of participants who visit booths set up by the local sponsors.

It was a very special day. I was heartened by the thousands of individuals, stretched out over several city blocks, who came to participate. At the starting line were the five-kilometer runners/walkers, followed by those doing three kilometers. George and I took our places among people of all ages, from babies in strollers to seniors in wheelchairs. Some wore special T-shirts displaying their support for a cancer cure. Pink was the dominant color, proudly stating: "I am a survivor." Many participants had posters pinned to their backs stating that they were walking in honor or memory of a friend or loved one. My sign said that I was walking "in honor of me—twelve years." What an emotional experience! George and I were visibly moved and frequently held hands as we walked with an estimated eleven thousand people. On completing the walk, each participant was given a "Race for the Cure" T-shirt. Survivors were given a pink shirt and cap. I wore mine with pride.

I believe there is a unique energy and bond created among strangers who share knowledge, hope, and understanding. The Wellness Community, Hope and Cope, and Gilda's Club (in memory of comedienne Gilda Radner, who died of ovarian cancer many years ago) just to name a few, are dedicated organizations available in many cities. They afforded me a chance to meet wonderful and caring people who understood what issues, we, as survivors, face every day.

*   *   *   *   *

I am completing this story while on vacation. George and I are on board a Princess Cruise ship, somewhere in northern Europe. We had flown to London first, where we discovered that my luggage was lost, but were reassured by the airline that it would soon follow. It is now one week later, ports have come and gone, and my suitcase still has not been found. How am I reacting to this major inconvenience? No problem. When put into perspective, it's just a little bump.

My roller coaster ride is over. I am in control again. I am a thirteen-year survivor!

*   *   *   *   *

One year later . . .

We enjoyed a wonderful winter in Florida. My health and renewed energy allowed us to participate in stimulating university courses, cultural events, and physical activities.

I am free of pain. There is residual tingling in my fingers, but sometimes it is so minimal I hardly notice it. I play the piano again and paint. George and I have begun traveling more. A spring cruise took us to Spain and Portugal. And there was a summer cruise through the Baltic Sea, with ports-of-call in Sweden, Denmark, Finland, Estonia, Poland, and St. Petersburg, Russia. I look at the world these days with new eyes—with a whole new appreciation for all that I've been so lucky to see and enjoy. Our plan is to return to Australia within the next year and resume the trip we abandoned three years ago.

I am *living* with cancer and enjoying *every day*!

Lorna continues to live with cancer after learning it has also metastasized to a lung. She travels to Memorial Sloan-Kettering in New York, where she receives ongoing treatment. Lorna and her husband still enjoy an active lifestyle together.

Alice Rollo

was born and raised in North Carolina. Happily married for forty-two years, she and her husband have three children, four grandchildren, and two step-grandchildren. No stranger to cancer, Alice has a strong family history of the disease and has lost several close relatives to it. Before her own bout with cancer, Alice was always a very private person, but now freely shares her cancer experience in order to help others. Alice knows the importance of annual checkups and routine mammograms; she spends her days working in the front office of a busy medical practice giving other women just such advice. She feels she could not have made it through her ordeal with the disease were it not for the loving support of her family and her strong faith in God. When not working, Alice enjoys church activities, sewing, scrapbooking, and spending time with her grandchildren.

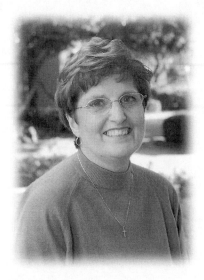

DIAGNOSIS PROFILE

Age at diagnosis:	60 years old
Family history:	Sister
Symptoms:	None—abnormal mammogram
Surgery:	Stereotatic core biopsy
	Lumpectomy
	Mastectomy
	TRAM flap reconstruction (right)
	Reduction (left)
Biopsy results:	Ductal carcinoma in situ (DCIS)
	Infiltrating ductal carcinoma
	Stage: 1
	Tumor size: 0.7 cm.
	Nodes: 24 negative
	Grade: 1
	Estrogen receptor low positive
Hormonal therapy:	Tamoxifen
	Pre-diagnosis: 14 years of HRT
Complications:	Lymphedema

Life is what happens to you when you're making other plans.
—Betty Talmadge

Home for the Holidays—
with Cancer

ALICE ROLLO

Christmas has always been my favorite season of the year. I love the music, decorating my house, sending and receiving cards, shopping for the perfect presents, and then watching everyone open their gifts. When our children were young, on Christmas Eve we would sit around the tree, and read the Christmas story and sing holiday songs. On Christmas Day, my husband, John, and I would eagerly get on the floor and play with our son and two daughters and all their new toys. Now that they are adults, we try to be with our grandchildren in the same way we once were with our kids. All through the years, I never dreamed that my precious holidays would one day be cruelly shattered.

I always had mammograms twice a year, in June and December. Ever since my sister was diagnosed with breast cancer in 1985, I began seeing a breast surgeon regularly. Not only did I have a mammogram every six months, my wonderful doctor would always get a second opinion. Therefore, I never considered any mammogram "routine."

On that fateful December day, I knew things were not as they should be. The mammography technician took me back five different times for more views, which was a dead giveaway that something was suspicious. There was a long wait, and during it, I started to sense that my results were not good.

Finally, the radiologist called me into his office and explained that I had "changes" in my right breast and recommended I have a needle biopsy. Apparently there were two questionable spots detected on the mammogram. He went on to tell me that 90 percent of the women who have biopsies have negative results. "That means 10 percent have positive results," I said. Plus, I had a strong family history of cancer. I was concerned.

I work in the front office at Roswell Obstetrics/Gynecology. My office Christmas party was that evening. I was in no mood for it. I just wanted to stay home and have a "pity party." However, John insisted that we go, and we did. It was so hard to smile and pretend that I was having a good time, that nothing was wrong, when my insides felt like jelly.

A week later, I had the stereotactic core biopsy. Not a good experience. The hospital was having problems with their new equipment, and I was kept waiting for over an hour while two repairmen worked on the machine—not exactly confidence inspiring. Waiting for those results was the longest week of my life.

There were only two people in my office who knew what I was going through. I have always been a very private person; therefore, I was not ready to share what was happening with everyone. As I expected and feared, the biopsy result was positive for cancer. For whatever reason, the radiologist had done the biopsy on only one of the two spots and that spot was "carcinoma in situ." I have no idea why he did not biopsy both spots.

Since I have always been a master at hiding my emotions and I didn't want to spoil anyone's Christmas, I decided not to tell my family. I wanted everyone to have a wonderful holiday without worrying about me. I do not believe John fully understood at that point that I had cancer, mainly because I used the term "neoplasm" (abnormal growth of tissue) instead of cancer.

Learning that I had cancer hit me hard. I was not shocked, mind you—my family and my husband's were riddled with cancer. I had an aunt and uncle who both had colon cancer. I had a sister who was a breast-cancer survivor for fifteen years. But she was also a heavy smoker and eventually died of lung cancer. I lost my mother to liver cancer four months prior to my diagnosis. Two months earlier, John's brother lost his seven-year battle against cancer, and his mother, too, lost her life to the disease. I was no stranger to the suffering and devastation of cancer and the early loss of beloved family members. I thought, now I might be one of them—what a way to start the New Year! I did feel fortunate that the cancer was detected early and that I had a loving husband and family, not to mention a great doctor. But I could not have made it through this period without my faith in God.

I felt a lot of anxiety the day before my lumpectomy. The fear of the unknown had taken over. The day of the surgery I was still trying to convince myself that this was not happening to me and that *someone* had made a huge mistake—I was in a state of denial. I will never forget arriving at the Breast Cancer Center and seeing the word *cancer* on the sign, in huge, bold letters. That was when it really hit me that I had the disease.

The day after surgery was a bad one. The pain medication caused a terrible headache, dizziness, light-headedness, and severe nausea. I spent most of the day throwing up. I also had a lot of swelling and pain in my breast. Though the lumpectomy was over, my nightmare was just beginning. My doctor had tried calling me at home, but I was unable to reach the phone before it stopped ringing, which ended up being a blessing in disguise. He reached me the next day at work, however, and informed me that my pathology report was worse than he had expected. One spot was "carcinoma in situ" but the other spot was "invasive." He had scheduled me for a mastectomy the following week! And he wanted me in his office with my husband the next day. The news was too overwhelming. I immediately fell apart. By some miracle, when I got off the phone with the doctor, John, who was out of town, was on the other line. The news quickly spread through my office and somehow I made it through the day. I drove home and there was John, pulling into the driveway at the same time I was.

The next morning at work was extremely rough. People who had just found out about the mastectomy were stopping by my desk to give me a hug. They wanted to talk about it, but I was unable to discuss any of it—I still hadn't accepted what was happening to me. The night before, I had even experienced a couple of panic attacks.

My surgeon, Dr. A., was wonderful at my preoperative appointment. I had made a list of questions, but his explanation was so thorough that I never even had to ask any of them. He knew me well, and he knew that I understood medical terms, but he also explained everything to John in layman's terms. He encouraged me not to hold my feelings inside, but to let them out.

Following my pre-op appointment, I basically cried for twenty-four hours. I was angry that the radiologist had not biopsied both spots. If he had, I would have had one less surgery to go through. Not only was I upset about having a mastectomy and not knowing what treatment I would need, if any, but two very important weddings were coming up: my son was getting married in one month and my daughter in four months. John got totally angry with me for worrying about the weddings, but they meant so much to me—I didn't have time to be sick, let alone have cancer!

I got angry, too. And I questioned my faith. I felt that I was handling the situation very badly; I should have been stronger. I talked with one of the ministers at my church who had been through his own battle with cancer and could relate to my feelings. He assured me that there was nothing wrong with my faith, but that I was hurting and it was all right to be scared, to feel weak, and to cry. He reminded me of the shortest Bible verse, "Jesus wept." Even Jesus cried when He was hurting. I took great comfort in the minister's words. I could almost feel my strength and courage returning right then. I had many calls that night and I knew that there were a lot of people praying for me. A peace and calmness settled over me. I still was unhappy about the cancer and the impending mastectomy, but I knew then that I would make it.

When I went shopping for a dress for my son's wedding, the sales clerk asked me what color the bride's mother was wearing. I told her I did not know, I did not care, and it did not matter. She probably thought that I was not thrilled about the wedding, but in truth, I was so looking forward to it. Then, as I tried on dresses, the saleswoman said something about my right breast being larger than my left and asked me if I had considered wearing a minimizer. I *was* wearing a minimizer. I just could not bring myself to tell her that the breast was swollen because I had had a lumpectomy the previous week, and I was going to have a mastectomy the next week. I imagined her telling the other clerks after I left that she had "just waited on a total bitch."

At this point, we had told only one of our three children about my breast cancer: my unmarried daughter who lived nearby—we talked on a daily basis. I had thought when I first had the lumpectomy that I would be all right and could wait until after my son's honeymoon to tell him. I was planning to tell my other daughter after my son's wedding. Well, never plan! My son-in-law took the news extremely hard since he had lost both his parents to cancer. And he took it upon himself to tell my brother and sister for me because I could not tell them. We had been through so much with my mother.

On the day I was scheduled to have my mastectomy, after my morning shower I stood in front of the mirror and cried. I was looking at two breasts, but I knew the next time I stood there I would have only one breast. It was devastating.

Even though I was upset over losing my breast, I went into surgery with total peace. There were so many people praying for me, and I knew that no matter what the outcome, I would be all right. God had never promised that I would not have problems, but He did promise that He would always be there. As I was wheeled into the operating room, I knew He was carrying me in His arms.

Surgery went very well. The modified radical mastectomy that Dr. A. performed removed the breast tissue, muscles surrounding the breast tissue, and nearby lymph nodes. He did not recommend reconstruction at the time of the mastectomy surgery because he did not know what I was facing. He did not know whether or not I would need chemotherapy or radiation therapy. Delaying reconstruction allowed the surgical wound to heal completely, so the reconstruction does not compound possible post-mastectomy healing problems. I remember waking up in the recovery room, and reaching up to feel my breast. It was so flat. I had gone into the hospital feeling like a complete woman, but I was leaving the hospital feeling like half a woman. I asked John how he felt about having a one-breasted wife. He got very annoyed. "I did not marry you for your breasts," he said.

After only a twenty-three-hour stay in the hospital, thanks to an unfortunate insurance company rule, I was released and sent home. Women who have just had such a traumatic operation should, I believe, remain longer in the hospital.

I had three phone calls after my surgery, from my son-in-law, my son, and my minister. I have been told that I said to my son-in-law, "I feel fine, I'm on pain pillows." I told my son in a high-pitched voice, "I'm fine, really I'm fine." No one will tell me exactly what I said to the minister; just that they are sure he talks to a lot of people who have just had surgery and are on pain medication.

Dr. A. was leaving on his vacation in two days and had requested the pathology results. The night before he left, he called to say that the pathology report showed another spot that had been removed, and that the mammogram had not detected, was also invasive. The good news was that the lymph nodes came back clear. Praise the Lord! Needless to say, I was elated. I got off the phone crying, but this time with tears of joy and relief.

I work with a wonderful and close-knit group of people. They had made me a "sunshine basket" with a gift for every day for two weeks, and the first thing I would do each morning was to open a gift. The love and concern of everyone was overwhelming.

It was about a week after surgery when I got the drains taken out that I first saw what my chest looked like with only one breast. I wish someone had warned me. The doctor almost had to peel me off the ceiling. What a horrible scar! In the mirror I saw a normal breast on one side, and on the other, a gruesome reminder of my surgery. My incision was different than most mastectomies since I already had two incisions from the lumpectomy. The mastectomy incision had to be made at a different angle, creating more scarring than is typical. And now, I would see it every time I undressed.

My children kept telling me how much they loved me, and my son-in-law called every day for a month. A time of crisis really wakes you up; it changes your way of thinking and reorganizes your priorities. Suddenly, every moment is precious and you are thankful for each day.

I do not know how I managed, but two weeks after my surgery, I made my granddaughter her flower girl dress. I had planned on making it before I was diagnosed with cancer. After all, I had waited a long time for my son to find that special person, and I had told him not to let her get away. It took me three times longer than usual to make the dress, but my doctor said it would be good therapy, and he was right.

A few weeks after surgery I found myself feeling very depressed, which was out of character for me. Not only had I lost a breast, I could no longer take the hormones that I had been taking for four-teen years. Naturally, I started having hot flashes and could not sleep. My best sleep had always been on my right side, and now with one breast missing, it was difficult to sleep on my side. I was not bal-anced, plus my right shoulder was bothering me a great deal. I did not have a chance to heal from the first surgery before I had the sec-ond. I did not want to go anywhere. I was lopsided and felt that everyone could see that, even though I was wearing big, loose shirts. I practically felt like a freak.

About that time, in the comic strip *Funky Winkerbean*, the char-acter Lisa had breast cancer and was having some of the same reac-tions that I was experiencing. Apparently, the creator of the comic strip had a close relative with breast cancer. In one of the strips, the husband asks if there's anything he can do, and Lisa answers, "I just want to be alone! I'm disfigured, exhausted, going bald, and gaining weight!" I was not going bald or gaining weight, but I could certainly relate to being disfigured and exhausted. In another strip, Lisa says, "Sometimes it takes a diagnosis like cancer to make you realize how beautiful the rain can be!" Another one had Lisa's friend say, "Normal isn't as normal as it once was!" And still another showed her going to the oncologist for the first time and saying, "Last year I couldn't even spell the word *oncologist!*"

I was very nervous about getting the surgical staples taken out. I was so certain it would hurt that I took pain medication before going to the doctor. It never occurred to me that the incision was still numb. While waiting for the doctor, I heard him talking to another patient who was going to need chemotherapy. It was another reminder to me how fortunate I was.

I had a temporary breast form that the American Cancer Society had sent me, and I was wearing it until my incision healed. Although I had it anchored, it still kept riding up. It was uncomfortable and was always moving out of place, and I self-consciously believed that everyone was looking at my crooked boob!

I went back to work too soon, after only three weeks. I know now that I should have waited longer before going back, not only for my body, but for my emotional healing as well. Everyone kept checking on me and telling me not to push myself, but I was not going to let a mastectomy sidetrack me. It did, however, slow me down. I had to take long lunch hours and leave work early.

It is traumatic for a woman to sit in front of a full-length mirror and try on a breast prosthesis. Since I had a very large bust, the prosthesis felt extremely heavy. However, wearing it did make me feel more like a whole woman. Still, I could no longer wear anything sleeveless or with a low neckline.

We had a friend from church whose mother was a seven-year breast-cancer survivor and was now considering reconstruction. Apparently, my husband told our friend that after my mastectomy, I would have reconstruction. However, I did not want to discuss it with anyone. Our friend told John not to push the issue, that I had already been through enough and it had to be my decision, not his. At that time, I could not even consider reconstruction. I had already been through two surgeries—I was tired, sleep deprived, and my whole body constantly ached. My right shoulder was particularly painful, and no matter how much I did my exercises, I could not raise my arm very high. I was so tired of hurting.

A month after my mastectomy, I was able to fly to Texas for my son's wedding—a team of wild horses would not have been able to stop me! My sister and my daughter and her family flew out from North Carolina, and other relatives came from South Carolina, plus my younger daughter and future son-in-law were there. On the night of the wedding rehearsal, my son-in-law put his arm around me and asked me which breast had been removed. He had been looking but could not figure out which one it was. Bless his heart. My sister felt the fake breast, then felt the real one to see if she could tell the difference. She could not.

It was a beautiful wedding, and I was grateful to be there. My son and his bride had wanted to cancel the lighting of the unity candle because they thought it would be too much for me, but I wouldn't let them. I have to admit that the trip totally wiped me out; I was a lot weaker than even I had realized.

The sister of a friend of mine called me one day at work to talk. She'd had a mastectomy ten years earlier and she understood all the feelings and emotions I was going through. I told her how upset I had been that morning because I could not put my necklace on and that I had just sat down and cried. She assured me that all my feelings were normal and things would improve.

Being without my estrogen therapy didn't help matters. I had hot flashes day and night and was not sleeping. I had mood swings and would cry for no reason at all. Up to this point, I felt I had done rather well, but I guess the lack of hormones was just kicking in. When I told my husband that I did not know what was wrong with me, he said, "Alice, you have had two major surgeries."

I do not believe John realized just how tired and depressed I was at this time. He traveled a lot and was only home on the weekends, so he didn't see me at my lowest. I never complained, and since I was good at hiding my emotions, he simply did not know.

I began a journal and in it I wrote:

I will never be the same. I'm still Alice but Alice only has one breast. Alice lost a breast to cancer. The day I found out that I had cancer changed my life forever. Every single day is precious. Every day I thank God that I am alive. There are so many that are not as lucky as I am. There are many going through chemo, radiation, and for some it is too late for even that.

Going to the oncologist for the first time was traumatic. I had always been a healthy person, and didn't go to the doctor often. Suddenly, I had all kinds of doctors and had an appointment with one every week. My husband did not want me to go alone, so he arranged his schedule in order to accompany me.

My oncologist assured me that nothing indicated that I would need chemotherapy or radiation. He recommended tamoxifen, in view of the estrogen-positive result in at least one of my biopsies, and as a means to reduce recurrence of breast cancer, risk of metastasizing, and protection of bone and cardiovascular systems. Since I had had a hysterectomy years earlier, endometrial cancer was not an issue. A major blessing, believe me.

A few weeks later, I received a call from the American Cancer Society. They wanted to know if I would mail envelopes to my neighbors for the annual cancer drive, and I immediately said yes. I carefully wrote a letter telling about my cancer, lumpectomy, and mastectomy. I felt that if I informed everyone of my own personal experience, people would be more likely to make a donation. Was I ever wrong! I was very disappointed and even a bit hurt when no one responded.

I had been through so many changes in my life in such a short period of time. Not being able to take the hormones gave me mood swings, hot flashes, night sweats, sleep deprivation, and I was not able to wear certain clothes. Every night when I took my bath, I had to carefully wash my fake breast since prostheses are very expensive. I was taking a bunch of vitamins and other medicine I had never taken before. I had been a person who only took hormone replacement and occasionally something for a headache. I had "sticker shock" the first time I paid for the tamoxifen.

When I saw my surgeon again he assured me that I was healing very well, but he thought I should be able to raise my arm higher. I told him that my shoulder would not let me. He thought I probably had bursitis in the shoulder, gave me something for the pain and said that if it was not better in a week, I would need to see an orthopedic specialist. Just what I wanted—another doctor!

I was beginning to think about reconstruction. I did not like wearing the heavy prosthesis, but I also was not too keen on having another surgery. I just wasn't ready for it, I guess. Partly because I had to attend to my shoulder first. I had slipped in my house one morning, which resulted in excruciating shoulder pain. Off to the orthopedic doctor I went. An MRI revealed that I had extensive adhesions, cartilage damage, and inflammation—all from an injury several years earlier. Basically, my shoulder was frozen. The trauma of my two back-to-back surgeries and the times my arm was immobile had exacerbated the already bad condition. I was scheduled for yet another surgery. Only it had to wait for several weeks—spring break was coming up, and I did not want to leave my office manager in a bind—a number of people were taking vacations. Waiting to have the surgery was pretty unbearable; I was in constant and ever-increasing pain.

I was having a hard time finding something to wear because everything had to button in front. Undressed, I looked like a freak, which upset me. I knew that I was very fortunate, but I was not able to control how I felt on the inside. There were days when it was so hard to go to work and put on a happy face, days when I did not want to leave my house. And I found that the least thing would start me crying.

John very much wanted to retire and to relocate, but I did not want to move and leave my doctors. They were my lifelines, my security blanket, and my husband did not understand that. Maybe someday I would change my mind, but I did not foresee that happening in the near future. Insurance was also a consideration. I was on John's insurance, so we really needed him to continue working. I am uninsurable since I have had cancer.

A friend of ours told us that his mother-in-law was dying of cancer. Hearing things like that upset me greatly. I was watching TV one night and there was a program on where a mother, with two children, was dying of cancer. I had to turn the TV off, and just sat and cried. Hopefully, some day I can hear the word *cancer* and not be scared.

Cancer was all around me. At the doctor's office where I worked, sometimes a patient would come for an appointment and she would comment, "The doctor is going to really fuss at me. I was due for a mammogram last year and haven't had it yet."

"*He* is not going to fuss at you; *I am*," I would say. Then, I would tell the woman that I was standing before her because my cancer was detected on a mammogram. I would go on to lecture about the need and importance of the mammogram—and who better to lecture her than someone who has had breast cancer? That always did it—the woman would go into her appointment and tell the doctor that he needn't bother lecturing her because I had already taken care of that. My having cancer resulted in a lot of people getting those mammograms that they had put off. At one of our offices, the women went several at a time for their mammograms. All the women at my husband's office made their appointments, too. I realized some good was finally beginning to come out of my nightmare.

I finally had arthroscopic shoulder surgery. Since I did not have lymph nodes on my right side, I had to constantly remind everyone at the hospital that the IV, blood pressure, etc. had to be on the left side. When my doctor was manipulating my arm and shoulder, he ripped my mastectomy incision in two places.

Two weeks after my shoulder surgery, my daughter got married. Thank goodness all the wedding arrangements had been made before I was diagnosed with cancer. My children and grandchildren were all here in Atlanta for the happy event. It was a gorgeous first of May—a perfect day for a perfect wedding. Once again, I was just grateful to be part of it.

Life itself had become even more precious to me than ever before. Things like the sunrise, sunset, laughter, and saying "I love you" became more important. I started calling my hot flashes "reminders" that I am still very much alive.

At the same time, I began obsessing over the fear that I would develop cancer in another part of my body. Or worse yet, pass it on to my two daughters and my beautiful granddaughter. This is not the legacy I wanted to leave them.

Slowly, and in small stages, optimism started to replace pessimism, and when I entered my first Relay for Life race, I began to feel inspired. Meeting twenty- and thirty-year survivors helped me a great deal, but seeing the many children who were cancer victims was hard to take. My husband and daughter were among the hundreds who lined the track to cheer us on as we made our victory lap. I was very choked up and cried the entire lap.

I continued to consider reconstruction. I figured that I had already had three surgeries; why not one more? I had not told John that I was even considering the surgery, and he had not mentioned it since our friend had told him to ease off that subject.

The wife of one of my husband's coworkers had a lumpectomy and, like me, two weeks later had a mastectomy. We talked quite often. I had already been there, and I understood how she was feeling. There was a big difference though; my husband would talk openly about the breast cancer. Her husband did not want to discuss it at all. I believe that is why she called me so often.

One of my coworkers was leaving, and the other women wanted to have a sleep-over party for her. I decided I could not go to it. I explained to the hostess that I had a difficult enough time removing my fake breast in front of my family, I certainly wasn't going to remove it in front of other people! I may not even have had to do so, but just the possibility was too much for me to handle. When I wore the prosthesis, I felt like a whole person. Once I took it off, I felt like a freak.

One day my daughter and I were shopping in a department store and discussing reconstruction. A salesclerk overheard our conversation and mentioned that two people she worked with had reconstruction and they looked great. It is amazing how many women have had breast cancer.

Two things that were greatly concerning me about the reconstruction were how much work I would miss and the fact that I would not be able to raise my arm above my head for several weeks. I was afraid my shoulder would freeze up again. It had also been a very expensive year; therefore, I was extremely concerned about the cost of this surgery.

Two months after I finished physical therapy for my shoulder, I left my orthopedic's office for the last time and called a plastic surgeon for an appointment. I had read a lot about reconstruction and discussed it a lot at work, but suddenly I was nervous. I knew that I wanted to have the surgery, not for my husband, but for me. I knew that it would make me feel better about myself. But facing the unknown again was frightening. However, God had seen me through everything else, so I knew He would see me through yet another surgery.

I fell in love with the plastic surgeon when I met him. He made me feel comfortable and relaxed. He also told me I was not a candidate for an implant because my incision was not the normal kind for a mastectomy. That was fine with me because I did not want an implant. He told me that I would need the free flap TRAM, but he would also need to do a reduction on the other breast because I did not have enough stomach fat to make a matching breast. In this operation, excess skin and fat from the lower abdomen are transferred to the mastectomy site and used to sculpt a new breast. This sounded great to me. I had always wanted to have a breast reduction, and now I was going to have a tummy tuck, too!

It was August and I set the surgery up for December. All the cancer walks were coming up in September and October, and I did not want to miss any of them. I also was waiting until after Thanksgiving so I would not mess up anyone's holiday. However, after a sleepless night, I called and changed the surgery date to September. I finally realized that it was time I did something just for me, to put *me* first for a change.

One night about a week later, I had just taken a shower and was standing in front of the mirror when I noticed a lump on my chest! It was located beside my incision. Needless to say, I panicked. I did not sleep well that night.

The next day I was in the surgeon's office. Dr. A. said it was probably a cyst, but he did a needle biopsy to be certain. I did not tell John because I did not want him to worry. I also was not going to tell anyone at my office, but I realized that I needed support. I knew God would carry me through this crisis as He had everything else. I finally told John and he reacted with great concern. I was scared, jumpy, and sick to my stomach until the biopsy report came back. Negative! There was a celebration at my office. Of course, everyone at the office had offered their stomach for the reconstruction surgery still to come.

A week before my reconstruction, my surgeon removed the lump. He felt that it had decreased in size, but I thought it was the same. I was under a local anesthetic while he removed it, so I did not feel anything. But I could *hear* him cutting the tissue. Just the night before at my support group, several of the women were talking about having their ports removed and being able to hear the cutting.

Maybe we should have all brought a favorite piece of music and a cassette player with us.

During my preoperative appointment, the plastic surgeon drew all over my chest with a bright blue magic marker. It was one doctor's visit I actually enjoyed. At last I was about to have a surgery that would make me feel good about myself.

When I awoke from the surgery I couldn't wait to look at my breast, which, by the way, did not have a nipple yet—that would come later. I was expecting to be covered with bandages, but all I had were steri-strips (a clear tape). I could now see both breasts; one, newly reconstructed, the other, reduced for a perfect match. It was totally amazing and beautiful! I had three drains and was on morphine so I was not feeling too much pain. And although it was difficult to get up off the bed and sit down, it was worth it. The plastic surgeon said there was a very slight flaw, a tiny speck of my hysterectomy scar was now on the new breast, but I would never have noticed it if the plastic surgeon hadn't mentioned it.

One night in the hospital I was having a hard time falling asleep, so one of the nurses stood by my bed and we talked for an hour. She kept telling me that I had the best breast she had ever seen. I had to agree that the plastic surgeon had done a remarkable job. And on top of that, I now had a flat stomach for the first time in twenty years!

Recovery had its difficulties. I moved very slowly, and was not able to stand up straight, and had to sit in a chair to take a shower. Several days after I was home, as I was preparing for bed one night, I was shocked to see that there was bleeding from my breast. I thought I had pulled a stitch. It turned out that someone had forgotten to inform me that I should expect some drainage for several days.

My wonderful sister took care of me again, this time for two weeks. I slept with five pillows, two under my head, one on my right side, one under my knees, and one for my stomach in case I had to cough. Standing up straight remained a problem for a while, and I could not bear to wear anything tight-fitting around my waist. So my wonderful husband went shopping and bought several loose-fitting, yet stylish, outfits for me. I also purchased a couple pairs of overalls that I still love to wear.

I was finally able to go shopping for a bra. Guess where I went? Victoria's Secret! I had never been able to shop there before, but now after the breast reduction and the reconstruction, I could buy one of those outrageously sexy bras! I shopped till I dropped.

I returned to work after five weeks, and once again worked shorter hours until my body would let me do otherwise. "Superwoman" now had limited strength, and when I got tired, which was often, my stomach pulled. At night I would come home and collapse in my lounge chair and not want to get up.

At one of my support group meetings, a psychologist who works only with cancer patients explained to us that it usually takes about two years before we stop letting cancer rule our lives. Cancer was on my mind daily, and so this revelation was particularly meaningful to me.

There was also a woman at that meeting who had just completed her chemo treatments. She told us that no one ever sees her without her wig, not even her husband or children. She said she always went into a closet to put her wig on. She also told the group that she acts as if everything is great, no matter how bad she feels. The psychologist shook her head and said that this was a very unhealthy way to cope because you do not always feel good and your family *should* know when you are having a bad day. Apparently, the woman couldn't cope with this advice—she never came back to another meeting, and I have often wondered what happened to her.

The anniversary of my biopsy arrived. What a year it had been! However, in that year I had made many new friends and grown closer to God. I had so many things to be thankful for—and I was.

Christmas was a joyful holiday again. I relaxed and took special pleasure in the season and being with my grandchildren. As far as I knew, I was cancer-free. I realized I had been through some rough times, but it could have been a lot worse. Now I truly understood the saying: "God does not give us any more than we can handle."

The following February, I had the second stage of the reconstruction, the nipple-areola. It was also necessary for the surgeon to trim the new breast just a little. This surgery was outpatient, and I was given the choice of being awake or asleep. I chose to be asleep because I *never* wanted to hear the cutting of tissue again. The surgery went well, and I returned to work the next day.

I wore bandages for three weeks, and then came my postoperative exam and the unveiling of my new nipple. The nurse warned me that it would look large and a little funny. She was right—it was overly large and it did look strange, but the plastic surgeon assured me that the size would decrease.

Soon afterward I had an appointment with my oncologist. I asked, "How do we know that I don't have cancer somewhere else in my body?" His answer was, "You don't." He told me to become aware of my body, and if I feel that something isn't right, to simply have it checked out.

My breast seemed to be a frequent topic of conversation in my office, and so, one day, a new employee who didn't know that I had had cancer, a lumpectomy, a mastectomy, and reconstruction, asked me why I would have a reduction and breast lift at my age. I replied, "Now wouldn't I look strange to have one young, perky breast while the other breast was headed south?" That was the end of that conversation.

My second Relay for Life came around—and what a night it was. The weather was cold, windy, and threatening rain, but everyone's spirits were high. We danced and sang while waiting for the festivities to begin. The speaker, who was also a survivor, spoke about how he felt when he found out he had cancer. It was how I had felt:

numb and in shock. I never felt bitter, but I was numb. We all acknowledged how thankful we were to be alive and to be able to take that victory lap.

About two and a half months after getting the nipple-areola, I was able to have the final stage in the reconstruction process—color tattooing of the nipple-areola. Everyone at my office knew I was getting my tattoo and, of course, they wanted to see it. I'm afraid I was too modest—there was no way I was going to show them—even though I had told them I would. John purchased a beautiful rose tattoo from Party City. The day I went to work after the bandages were removed, everyone begged to see the tattoo so I finally revealed my rose.

I convinced one girl at work that it was a real tattoo, and, in fact, it did look real. She was aghast and couldn't believe I would "do something like that." I told her that my new breast was my beautiful rose. I never confessed to her that it was not real, and to this day she still thinks I have a rose tattoo on my breast. By the way, my lovely rose lasted for about a week.

My new breasts were doing just fine, thank you, and looked better than ever. Which is partly why, a few months later, I did something modest ol' me would *never* have done before. A patient was in our office one day and said she had just been diagnosed with breast cancer. She was distraught, frightened, depressed, shocked, and not dealing with these all-too-familiar feelings very well. One of the nurses asked me to talk to her. I prayed that God would put the right words in my mouth. Then, as I was speaking to her, I realized what she needed was to see the proof of what I was saying. So I showed her my reconstructed breast. Doing this and explaining everything I went through gave this woman more hope, encouragement, and probably did more to assuage her fears than anything or anyone else, including a doctor, could have said or done. It was then that I thought that perhaps God had allowed me to have cancer so that I could help other people.

Mind you, there are still days when, just out of the blue, I will start thinking about my strong family history of cancer, and the fact that I had it, and it will start me crying. Hopefully, I can overcome that someday.

Unfortunately, my diverticulitis, which I had kept under control for four years, started acting up. One day at work I doubled over with a horrible, sharp pain in my abdomen. I managed not to let anyone know and made it through the day. Within the next week my gastroenterologist put me on strong antibiotics, a liquid diet, and scheduled me for a colonoscopy.

The procedure went well, and the results I prayed for came in— no cancer! But my colon would not behave, and two weeks before Thanksgiving, the doctor told me that I needed surgery. God was still trying to get my attention. And He succeeded.

Thanksgiving Day came and my children and their spouses and my grandchildren were all at my house. I had prepared a feast for my family, but all I was allowed to eat were mashed potatoes and a little turkey. It was very difficult to watch everyone else "pig out." I waited until my family finished their meal before I dropped the bomb that I was once again having surgery.

I managed to purchase and wrap all my Christmas gifts and address and mail all my Christmas cards in one week. And then I checked into the hospital and had fourteen inches of my colon removed. I was extremely fortunate. The pathology report showed that I had a perforation, but it had sealed itself off.

Two days after surgery, the doctor took me off oxygen and told the nurse to get me up a couple of times a day. The nurse helped me to my chair, and an aide came in with a clean gown and towels and told me that I needed to learn to take care of myself. What?! I had a tube in my nose that went to my stomach, a catheter, an epidural, an IV, and pulsating devices on my feet! Totally speechless, I stared at the aide. Thank goodness, my husband walked in at that moment and helped me.

Despite losing seventeen pounds and having been completely wiped out by the surgery, Christmas was a joyous occasion with my family, and once again the holiday was cause for grateful rejoicing.

So was January. I had been cancer-free for two years. What a glorious feeling that two-year mark was—one of the great milestones of my life.

Two years and two months after my mastectomy, I noticed swelling in my right arm. I had flown to Texas to see my new grandson, and one night when I was undressing, I noticed that my arm was swollen. I had hoped it was attributable to all the salty food I'd eaten that day. Unfortunately, that was not the case.

After returning from Texas, I put the swelling out of my mind. However, one day when I was shopping for a new dress, the right sleeve was a little tight, and I realized I had more swelling than I had thought. I knew immediately that I had lymphedema. *I could not believe I had something else wrong with me.* Not only did I have swelling in my arm; it was swollen under my arm and across my back. I told the therapists at the Lymphedema Center that I thought it was fat, but they told me to look in the mirror and see if I looked that way on the other side. I had to give up my pretty Victoria's Secret bras and buy not-so-pretty, wide-strapped ones. (My daughter was more than happy to take the Victoria's Secret bras off my hands.) I began therapy for my arm, which involved various exercises and the wrapping of my arm like a mummy.

I thought I had been doing everything to prevent this condition. However, I did not have a compression bandage on when I flew to Texas—a big mistake—but in all honesty the thought never occurred to me. All I was thinking about was holding my new grandchild. I did not realize that being right-handed and having had the lymph nodes removed from my right side may have increased my risk for developing this condition.

My husband was out of town when I went to therapy for the first time, and he had forgotten that I had an appointment. When he saw my arm he said, "What have you done now?" He arranged his schedule so he could attend a therapy session, where he learned how to move the fluid across my back and arm and how to wrap my arm. My therapist told me how lucky I was because many husbands do not want to get involved.

My surgeon was terribly upset that I had developed lymphedema; in fact, I believe he was more upset than I was. The way I felt about it was summed up perfectly by an encounter I had one day with an elderly woman in the supermarket. She asked what was wrong with my arm, and I explained what it was. I also told her that I could live with lymphedema, but I could not live with cancer. She wished me well and told me to keep up the good attitude.

Lymphedema is extremely inconvenient. I had to greatly reduce my sodium intake and give up some favorite foods that are high in salt, such as Chinese, Mexican, and Italian dishes that I love. I use a low-sodium cookbook now. Heat and humidity are very bad for the arm, so I do not take part in outdoor activities in the warm months. Repetitive movements against resistance are not good for the arm, so I had to give up vacuuming and mopping. However, John now does that for me, so all changes are not so bad! I always liked to take hot showers, but that is out. I have learned to use my computer mouse with my left hand, which was a real challenge. I have also learned to iron with my left arm, and that takes me much longer now. I cannot sleep on the affected arm; therefore, I sleep with a pillow on my right side to rest my arm on. In fact, I sleep with so many pillows that my husband calls them my "pillow farm."

I am still wearing the wrapping bandages on the arm, and that makes a lot of chores more difficult. There is a girl at work who is an athletic trainer at one of the local high schools, so she usually wraps my arm for me. But I have also found that a lot of people want to open doors, carry my packages, and show sympathy for me.

I am currently awaiting my custom-made compression sleeve. I will probably need to wear it all the time, but it should make some things easier and less uncomfortable to do. And one day, the sentinel node biopsy will be perfected as an alternative to axillary node dissection. When that happens, women will have much less chance of being disfigured by a swollen limb. One day.

*   *   *   *   *

My family was once again struck by cancer. My younger brother is currently undergoing chemotherapy for colon cancer. Out of the five of us children, three have had cancer. I pray that my older sister and brother will be spared.

In the meantime . . . life goes on, as it must. I've learned so much from my cancer experience. It has made me more compassionate, renewed my faith in God, and forced me to draw from an inner strength I never knew I had. It taught me to use my experience to help someone else, and that by doing so, I also help myself. Cancer has made me aware of any and every change my body goes through. It has taught me to stay well informed and to maintain a healthy lifestyle. To research surgeries, treatments, and medications. To question doctors and get second opinions. To never lose a sense of humor. To allow deep and painful feelings to surface and be shared with others. To think positively—it boosts the immune system and aids in the healing process. To write down observations, thoughts, and insights. And to appreciate the beauty that's all around us in nature, but above all, in those we love and cherish.

Alice recently celebrated five years of being cancer-free with a lavish night out with her husband. And, they are happily awaiting the arrival of their fifth grandchild. Although Alice's husband is now retired, she loves her job and continues to work.

Sheryl Siegel

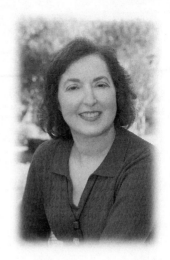

*worked in the travel industry for fifteen
years after earning a bachelor's degree in
biology in 1970. She then found her real
passion as a freelance photographer, and
during the mid-90s her work appeared in
such publications as* Newsweek *and the*
Atlanta Journal-Constitution. *She was
selected by the Atlanta Committee for
Olympic Games to photograph the 1996
Olympics. Community service is a priority
for Sheryl. She has been active in
President Jimmy Carter's Atlanta Project,*
*photographing various events to help low-income communities, and she
tutors reading at an elementary school near her home.*

DIAGNOSIS PROFILE

Age at diagnosis:	52 years old
Family history:	No knowledge
Symptoms:	Self-discovered lumps in both breasts
Surgery:	Core biopsy
	Bilateral mastectomy
	TRAM flap reconstruction
Biopsy results:	Infiltrating ductal carcinoma
	Microscopic multi-focal sites in both breasts
	Stage: 3
	Tumor size right breast: 3.5 cm. & 1 cm. satellite nodule
	Tumor size left breast: 2 cm.
	Nodes: 10 of 12 positive on right; none removed left
	Grades: 2 & 3
Chemotherapy:	Epirubicin, Cytoxan, 5-FU (5-Fluorouracil), Taxol
Radiation therapy:	18 of 24 treatments
Stem cell transplant:	High-dose chemotherapy
Hormonal therapy:	Tamoxifen
	Pre-diagnosis: 20 years of oral contraceptives
Complications:	Clot in chest port
Age at recurrence:	54 years old
Symptoms:	Burning in mid-back
Scan results:	Metastasis to spine and liver
	Stage: 4
Hormonal therapy:	Femara (taken off tamoxifen)
Radiation therapy:	14 treatments to spine
Chemotherapy:	Xeloda

Friendship is a guiding lamp, a door to understanding,
a window to the soul of self.

—Isabela Burani

The Worst—and the Best— Were Yet to Come

SHERYL SIEGEL

January, several years ago, was the worst month of my life. It was also the start of the most profound changes that have ever occurred in my life—I was being prepared for the woman I was to become.

I thought I had created change in my life since my father's death ten years earlier. I thought I was a completely different person from the quiet, shy girl who grew up lonely and afraid. I thought I had become a more open, giving person, who knew what she wanted out of life, who had discovered a talent and love for photography, and achieved lasting friendships. I became involved in community service to children, and with the help of a success coach, had created a stronger, more focused photography business. I signed my first twelve-month advertising contract. I knew where my life was going. I was on the road to happiness.

And then I hit a major detour: I discovered lumps in both my breasts, and they were growing. There was no history of cancer in my family, only heart disease. I felt healthy. I had never had anything other than a few childhood illnesses. I'd always assumed I would die of heart disease; cancer was never on my radar screen.

The lumps grew larger. I had never even had a mammogram, although my gynecologists through the years had always recommended one, starting at age forty. I saw all the commercials about self-exam and read articles about the increase of breast cancer, but I had a business to run and a life to lead—I felt safe. I never knew anyone who had had any form of cancer (so I thought!).

*   *   *   *   *

I led a life of desperate loneliness in my youth. When I was ten years old, my family moved from Memphis, Tennessee, to the small town of Birmingham, Alabama, to start a business. Uprooted from childhood friends and beloved family members, I felt adrift and unable to fit in. I envied my younger sister, Susan, who developed friendships right away. A stray cat I adopted became my source of comfort. School was a challenge for me socially—I made no friends. My father worked day and night at his new business. My mother found time to help him while caring for four children. I felt her absence, both physically and emotionally. Sitting on the back porch, holding my cat, I would cry in my loneliness.

By the time I became a teenager a few friendships had developed—I even had a boyfriend. Still dominated by fear and loneliness, all I desired was the love and attention of my parents and peers. How I wanted someone to just listen to me.

College was a whole new beginning for me. I was working toward my childhood dream of becoming a veterinarian. I did reasonably well in my classes and had a few friends, but still carried that scared, lonely girl with me.

Getting into vet school in the late '60s, when women were fighting for equal rights, was going to prove an impossible challenge. Although my grades were average, my belief in my dream was strong. But as I sat in front of the dean at my entrance interview, vying for one of the thirty available spots, he looked at me from behind his desk and said, "Why should I give you this spot when you'll just get married and quit?"

In disbelief I said, "I may get married someday, but I intend to work my entire life." I was not accepted. I left college with an undergraduate degree, but with no goals, and no idea of who I was or where I belonged. The loss of my dream threw me into a limbo that lasted more than twenty years.

I moved to Atlanta, Georgia, to start my life anew. I set up housekeeping with a roommate and went job hunting. When you don't know what you want to do, job hunting becomes a dart game. After several unsuitable jobs, I finally landed a position in the travel industry, which I loved. I also took up the joyous hobby of square dancing and slowly began to build a social life. There was even a new romance. DJ became my "guardian angel" and an important part of my life.

Still struggling with low self-esteem, the overwhelming loss of my father threw me into a deep depression. He was my "rock," the one person I had looked to for love and financial support. He had given me everything. My family members had their spouses to help them deal with their grief; I felt alone with mine. But my father's death was also a turning point in my life. Along with individual therapy, I joined my first support group: Codependents Anonymous (CoDa). My arduous journey out of a twenty-year limbo had begun.

CoDa brought many new friends and awarenesses. I learned to speak my truth and trust my gut. I was not alone. My faith in God deepened, along with my belief in the guiding spirits I called "angels." I learned that other people did, in fact, like me and even loved me for just being me. The love I had for myself and others that had always been hidden inside began to blossom. Therapy taught me how to cope with my fears and respond differently to the world around me, not as the scared, lonely girl I used to be, but as the strong, courageous adult I truly was.

Following my passion for photography, I faced more fears. I learned to interact with strangers, allowing them to see my soul through the lens of the camera. I learned to play, to see the world, and to be a part of the community.

My independent circles of friends grew—photographers, clients, networking groups, volunteers, support groups, and fellow square dancers. Each was a separate but vital part of my life as a photographer and community advocate.

*   *   *   *   *

After feeling lumps in my breasts, I went to see a gynecologist in January. My gut was telling me something was wrong—not an auspicious way to begin the new year. The doctor announced that both my breasts needed biopsies.

Mammograms, sonograms, needles, and doctors were new experiences for me. While waiting to hear from the radiologist who had done my biopsies, I continued to tell myself it could not be cancer.

On January 30, the phone rang as I sat alone at my computer. *Please let January end on a good note*, I prayed. Instead, I heard the words, "I'm sorry to tell you this, but you have cancer in both your breasts. Please call Dr. G., who is an oncologist, immediately to set up an appointment." Shock set in. Fear immediately followed. Confusion was next.

I knew I needed knowledge and a support group to help me cope with whatever lay ahead for me, starting with one terrifying diagnosis. I was told about The Wellness Community breast-cancer support group that met each Wednesday—the day before my first oncology appointment. Somehow I made it to Wednesday. I walked into the meeting room with my red notebook, and my life was forever changed.

It was a room filled with women, some with no hair, some young, some my age, some white, some black—all dealing with cancer. I got what I needed that day, which was information to prepare me for my oncology visit, and made new friends who knew what I was facing because they had been there. Several women approached me after the meeting and gave me their phone numbers, saying, "Please call."

Invited by Robin (whose story is also in this book), I joined the group for lunch. They talked in a new language—path reports, chemo drugs, treatments, and blood counts. Things I would all too soon learn about and become intimately familiar with. But for now, relationships were forming, family and friends were warmly discussed, and occasionally laughter broke out.

Armed with breast-cancer information from Dr. Susan Love's Web site and accompanied by my best friend Pam, I went to Dr. G.'s office the next afternoon. After filling out the medical paperwork, I was weighed, then my blood pressure, temperature, and pulse were taken. On to the lab for blood work. CBC—what did that mean? I was soon to learn all about my blood. Back in the exam room I sat on the table wrapped in the paper gown. Dr. G. came in, shook my hand and asked, "How are you doing? I'll examine you first and then we'll talk in my office."

Dr. G. was efficient and thorough as she felt my neck, breasts, underarms, and listened to my lungs and heart. "Get dressed, we'll talk," she said when the exam was over. I was still numb and in shock. I was very grateful for Pam's cool demeanor and presence of mind. She was able to absorb what I missed. Armed with my red notebook and a list of questions, I was ready to hear what was next.

I wrote in my journal that night:

Today I went to the oncologist. The news was not good: advanced stage breast cancer in both my breasts. Treatment would begin with four rounds of chemo followed by a double mastectomy, then more chemo. It should save my life, but will change me forever. I am scared, sad, and afraid of how I will look. I feel that sex will be gone forever from my life. I need strength and courage to see me through this. I need to love and nurture myself and focus all my attention on my body and spirit.

Chemo *before* the bilateral mastectomy was apparently necessary to first shrink the large tumors and, above all, destroy any cancer cells that might have already invaded nearby tissue—beyond the breasts themselves.

I listed my sources of love in my journal. I acknowledged my need to feel and heal. I asked God to help me make each day special. My team included everyone, starting with God, then me, then my family and friends, and my new family—the breast-cancer support community, all praying for my safe passage.

I committed myself to "living" that day. I surrendered my life into God's hands and guidance. I vowed to follow Him with all my strength, courage, and determination. In other words, to do whatever it took. I had my life and just for today I felt safe, loved, protected, healthy, fed, clothed, and financially provided for.

My family and friends gathered around me. They called, sent cards and e-mails as they helped me prepare for my changing life. A room in my house was cleaned for guests and family members who would be visiting and helping me—my old life was put away in storage. My journal kept me focused on my faith and love as I grew, changed, and accepted my new and different life—one with breast cancer in it.

That life now revolved around doctor visits, hospital tests, The Wellness Community's resources, support meetings, yoga, and new friends. My independent support circles came together. People from my business networks and volunteer activities called, sent cards, and offered their help. Offers to accompany me to chemo treatments, run errands, provide fun activities, and be physically present for me came without my asking. Hidden resources showed up through my friends, and I allowed myself to accept these gifts of love.

The preliminary testing, which included blood work, a bone scan, CAT scan, and heart tests, showed that the cancer was confined to my breasts and lymph nodes. Dr. G. and I discussed a new chemo drug called epirubicin that I had found on the Internet. Her research helped me feel comfortable with being her first clinical patient to try this treatment. My first chemo rounds included Cytoxan, 5-FU (5-fluorouracil), and epirubicin. Dr. G.'s expertise and her look-you-in-the-eye-and-tell-it-like-it-is attitude gave me the confidence to place my life in her hands.

People continued to show up from all corners and connections. My circles became intertwined, and my needs were provided for. God was working overtime on my behalf. I just kept walking and doing my job—making calls, asking for help, accepting what was offered, and letting go of the rest.

As I moved from the doing, the frightened feelings began to resurface, although the shock and numbness were easing. I felt alone, although I had all the loving support I needed by my side. Family, friends, doctors, and what I call "the loving spirits of the universe" showed me the way. They held my hand and prepared me for my journey. I accepted the frailty of my body, and the wholeness of my spirit and soul. I came to terms with my death. But until then, I would offer my life as an example of what goodness, courage, and love could be.

My faith guided me to doctors who were the perfect match for me. I followed my gut for guidance in all my decisions. I became grateful for a smile, a kind word from strangers, and a hug from a friend. Empowered by the loving support of all my communities, I heard over and over again how I had touched their lives, giving them strength and courage, just by being me. This was an extraordinary opportunity to see the impact I had made on the people in my life. Like the character George Bailey from my favorite movie *It's a Wonderful Life*, I was shown the power of one—enabling my soul the freedom to breathe.

My friend Devorah came with me to my first chemo treatment. She brought blankets, water, and ice to help combat any side effects. The nurse made sure the drugs did not injure my veins and slowed the process when my arm began burning. That night I took the anti-nausea drug Kytril. Knowing that each person responds differently to chemo, I did not want to be alone my first night, so another friend stayed with me—just in case.

The next day I was busy with phone calls and activities. I attended The Wellness Community breast-cancer support group to nurture my newly formed friendships. That night, feeling the effects of the chemo, I found eating rice helped relieve the nausea and settle my stomach.

Three days later, the nausea grew worse. I added bananas to my meals of rice and continued to take the anti-nausea drug. Friends came to visit or to stay over, but I still felt shaky and alone.

On the fourth day, I added Compazine, another anti-nausea drug. It created anxiety overload—I was climbing the walls and could not sit still. Once I took my daily anti-anxiety drug, I calmed down. I did not do *that* drug again. By the next day, I was ready to get back to my daily life.

Preparing for the most noticeable change, the loss of my hair, I purchased a wig and got my hair cut. But it did not really prepare me for the first time a handful of hair came out in my brush, about three weeks after my first chemo treatment. Hair was everywhere—on my pillow, the floor, in the shower. As the bald spots appeared, I started wearing caps, and then my wig. I felt ugly. I couldn't even look at my head, and kept it covered most of the time.

At my follow-up visit with Dr. G., I learned that my white cell count was very low. She prescribed Neupogen injections during the next cycle of chemo to help jump-start it. Not comfortable with injecting myself once a day for ten days I called Elaine, a neighbor and nurse, to help me.

The low white cell count affected what I could eat—no fresh fruits and veggies because of the possibility of bacterial infection. I took antibiotics as a preventive. I was losing weight and attributed it to my change in diet—or maybe it was from the treatment.

I learned more about my disease, the drugs used to treat it, and invaluable coping skills. Ann Brett, a member of my cancer support group, so aptly stated, "The learning curve for cancer is straight up." I felt luckier than most women, having learned about the various treatments and surgery options early on in my diagnosis. I was able to pick my poison and choose my surgeons based on firsthand experience.

Through recommendations I found a caring and compassionate surgeon to place a port in my chest that would access my veins for the chemo and blood draws. Dr. L. answered all my questions about the surgery and counseled my fears. With my hair now gone, the port would become part of my new body.

I reconnected with my long-time friend and former lover, DJ—I needed to feel loved, physically. I was about to face the loss of both my breasts, along with my body image. Although I was receiving wonderful love from my women friends, the physical love of a man was a major concern for me. I feared that the loss of my breasts would end my sexual life—I needed DJ's male presence. Sharing my deeply personal emotions with someone who knew and loved me made me feel safe. I needed to know that he would still be sexually attracted to me—bald, with no breasts. I also needed to know that love was not all about my body, but really all about me. I found out that he loved me, bald, scared, and weak—it made no difference to him how I looked.

The port surgery was scheduled the day before my second round of chemo. That treatment was supposed to be easier—it wasn't. Accompanied by my friend Jeri, I was hooked up to an IV and immediately felt pain and burning around my new port. To avoid potential problems, the IV was slowed down. As a result, the three-hour procedure took six and a half. Jeri stuck with me through it all.

The next evening another friend, Heather, came to stay overnight to help me, and Elaine started the Neupogen shots. The third day was really rough—and all my stomach could handle were bananas and juice. By the fourth day, I was feeling much better. I now had a pattern to help get me through the remaining two chemo treatments.

The burning I experienced around my port concerned Dr. L. He sent me immediately to the hospital radiology department, but after several extremely painful sticks to my chest, the radiology nurse could not access my port for the dye test to detect the problem. Dr. L. was summoned and came to the hospital. After one more painful stick, he checked the results and proclaimed that I was fine.

Chemo became easier with the port in place, and the use of Elma cream numbed my skin and prevented pain prior to the stick. Bananas and grapefruit juice got me through the night of my third treatment when I once again experienced nausea. I was becoming an expert on nausea control.

My life revolved around chemo treatments, doctor visits, blood checks, and ten days of Neupogen shots. What was normal? I didn't know anymore. Cancer had invaded my life. I maintained contact with friends inside and outside my cancer support network and ran my photography business when I was able to work.

So that I could celebrate Passover, the Jewish holiday of family and remembrance, with my family in Birmingham, my last treatment before surgery was moved up a day. My mother and siblings planned extra-special foods for the Seder dinner and extra meals that

I could bring home to eat during the eight-day holiday. It was my first visit with my family since my diagnosis. While preparing my own home for Passover, I wondered how I would manage. Ann, from my support group, offered to make some Passover veggies for me. As she continued to struggle with her own cancer treatments, she somehow found time to help me. I will never forget her generosity.

My mother was having trouble with the fact that her "little girl" had a life-threatening disease, but ironically, for the first time, I felt I was a real part of my family—loved and nurtured. They played an important role in my healing.

As the months passed, I learned more about lumpectomy versus mastectomy, reconstruction or not. Dr. L. continued to check my port and discuss my surgical options. The chemo shrunk my tumors, and I prayed that one of my breasts might be spared.

The fear of surgery and how it would affect my body was often overwhelming—the loss of my sex life and the possibility of lymphedema affecting my photography career weighed heavy on my mind. Talking with my support friends helped, but the final decisions rested with me. Could I deal with this new body? Being bald and coping with chemo and its side effects seemed easier than dealing with a complete body change.

It became clear that a bilateral mastectomy with TRAM reconstruction was my best choice—the full monty. It would rid me of the cancer, and I would learn to deal with the effects—one day at a time.

I also searched for answers regarding my renewed sexual relationship with DJ. I would need his help with the emotional trauma of my body changes after surgery. Would he still desire me sexually? Would I still desire him?

With my initial treatments behind me, I had a sonogram to determine the results of the chemo treatments. I also received my first Procrit shot to help me with the overwhelming tiredness I felt from my low red blood cell count. Surgery was delayed from late

May to early June as necessary appointments took longer than antic-ipated. I continued to pray for divine order.

I marched on, mustering my support troops. My sister, Susan, offered her help, so I asked her to come the first week after surgery to care for me. I arranged time slots (to help me through the first three weeks after surgery) with each of my siblings and relatives who had answered the call. I wanted everything arranged before the first surgical cut. A part of me needed the *illusion* of control to feel safe. It eased my fears about my physical well-being as I faced being unable to care for myself alone. I had always "done it alone" or believed that I had. Of course, no one really does anything alone—my angels always silently stepped in when needed. My strength and courage increased daily as I learned the lessons of compassion, trust, and faith.

DJ continued to visit and give me his emotional and physical love. As I struggled with my body image, bald and feeling ugly, he continued to show me that all he wanted was for me to be well and healthy again. Each time we made love I believed it would be the last time as a whole woman—it brought me great emotional distress. His assurance that he would walk this journey with me for as long as nec-essary got me through many lonely, fearful nights.

I met with my plastic surgeon, Dr. B., to discuss the reconstruc-tion procedure. Dr. B. was a kind and funny little pixie. He was also passionate about helping women retain their body image. He gave me a full description of the procedure, using diagrams and pictures. Most of my questions were answered before I even asked them. He talked about the abdominal surgery or "tummy tuck," saying, "And lots of women *pay* to have this done." I was entertained, educated, and energized—surgery was scheduled.

After an encouraging radiology report that my tumors had shrunk by half from the chemo treatments, my pre-op visit with Dr. L. went very well. After some discussion, we agreed that he would use the side cut, so I would not have a scar on the topside of my new breasts. He planned to take less lymph tissue from my left side than from the right, reducing my chances of developing lymphedema and enabling greater mobility of my left arm.

My first Tuesday night cancer support meeting brought the beginning of another close friendship. As I talked about my fears concerning the upcoming surgery, Gayle spoke of her bilateral mastectomy and implant reconstruction. We exchanged phone numbers, then she asked if I would like to see her breasts. As she lifted her shirt and bra, she must have noticed the change in my facial expression. As soon as I got home she called and asked, "Are you all right?" I said that I was shocked, not at the sight of her breasts, but at the realization that I would soon undergo the same surgery. She gave me emotional support as well as practical information that night: get lots of pillows, wear slip-ons to avoid having to bend over to tie your shoes, and be sure someone is with you for at least the first two weeks—maybe longer.

I looked for a place in the mountains to spend Memorial Day weekend. I needed a change of scenery, a place that would bring some serenity to my life. Patricia, one of my support group friends, agreed to join me, and off we went to a lovely mountain lodge in North Carolina.

The first evening there, as I sat rocking in a chair on our balcony facing the forest, I listened to the birds as sunset approached and felt at peace. The next morning we selected what was supposed to be a "moderate" hike—it was anything but.

Up the mountain took about an hour. The view was incredible and I lingered to draw peace and energy from the surrounding beauty. Patricia had begun to head down the other side. Alone, I started down a steep, rocky trail, fearful that I had somehow lost the right path. Continuing down, I struggled over rocks and slid down the mountainside looking for Patricia. Completely alone and scared,

I walked for what seemed like forever, but was probably only about thirty minutes, when two hikers came up the path. Relieved, I asked if they had seen Patricia and they said that she was not far ahead of me. I kept walking, sliding and climbing, expecting to see her at each turn. Other hikers came up the path and continued to encourage me. Finally, I saw Patricia. We had made the difficult journey down separately, but together.

The mountain hike on that perfect day represented my current life—and the life that I would have in the future. I had had a relatively easy walk up the mountain of life, and now I faced the steep, rocky trip down alone—yet not alone. When I reached the end of the trail, I would be joined in celebration by all my fellow travelers. At Patricia's urging, I picked up a stone as a memento of that incredible day.

I reflected in my journal about the mountain trip and about change. Standing still no longer served me. Each stop was just as beautiful, if not more so, as the last, and I needed to change in order to fully experience it.

* * * * *

The pre-op visit with Dr. G. included a simple port flush. The nurses could not get the flush to go in, so I was scheduled to go to the hospital ER the next morning. The ER that day was a study in miscommunication. After the nurse had painfully stuck me twice with no results, Dr. L. was called and I was sent to radiology for "another" dye test that revealed the port was cracked, which explained the problems I'd been having with it during the past few months. Dr. L. read the report and said that the port needed to be replaced, but it could be done during surgery. Meanwhile, I was advised to be careful; the tip could break off, causing more problems. I hated that port.

I asked DJ to come to the hospital the day of my surgery. He said nothing would keep him away. Our lovemaking had been very emotional. Would I ever again feel sexual? Would I feel *sexy*? *Goodbye breasts. This is the last time. Remember the feelings. Goodbye.*

I had a million things to do the day before the surgery. My mother and her friend Ken arrived midday so that I could drop off my car for repairs. That evening, after receiving many supportive calls wishing me well, I stood in the shower and said my final goodbyes to my breasts and to the cancer that had invaded them. I prayed that God would bless me with the strength and courage to handle the surgery. Change, not by choice, but by acceptance, filled my life. The sisterhood to which I now belonged showed me how precious life was and to live it to the fullest with love.

At 5:00 a.m. I drove with my mother and Ken to the hospital. With my mother at my side, I lay nude under a sheet in the pre-op area. Then DJ arrived—I was so happy to see him. Cold and scared, he kissed me and stroked my arm to warm me. We spent fifteen minutes alone, then he and my mother stayed by my side until they wheeled me into the operating room.

I don't remember much until I found myself in my room later that afternoon, still fuzzy from the anesthesia. I had a catheter, and my legs and feet were in something that kept the circulation going. I was propped up with pillows and couldn't move. I also could not see well without my glasses, which I had left in the car that morning. I spent a very uncomfortable night, and the private-duty nurse hired to help me had an "attitude" and was inattentive to my needs.

The next day's private-duty nurse was much more helpful, as I struggled to get in and out of bed. Non-stop visitors and phone calls brought so much love and support. I began feeling stronger. And, at long last my mother brought my glasses—I could see again! Dr. L. came by to check on me and brought welcome news. He did not remove *any* tissue from my left lymph area.

The unpleasant night nurse arrived with an even worse attitude. I was really glad when Sunday morning brought enjoyable visits with my family and friends. My brother Lennie drove in from Birmingham to see me. By that evening, I was able to move around a little easier.

Monday morning the first of my six drains was removed and the IV moved from my right arm to my new port. Pain pills replaced the IV morphine. On Tuesday, before leaving the hospital, another drain was removed. I decided to take a shower and got undressed. Although I felt relief that I had gone into surgery with two breasts and came out with two new ones, I still avoided looking at them, but I did notice that tape was covering the actual scars. I called the nurse, who put a chair in the shower stall and gave me a fresh gown and towel. She said to call if I needed any help.

Easing myself into the shower, I sat in the chair and adjusted the water temperature. Expecting the water to come out the hand-held spout, I was totally shocked when cold water poured from the showerhead, blinding me. Turning off the water, I attempted to dry myself. My mother had arrived, and I called her for help. She dried my back. I wondered if she was reminded of when I was a baby, as I stood there nude and helpless. My clothes would not accommodate my drains and bandages, so I was offered a hospital gown to wear home.

With my mother's cotton robe draped over my shoulders and wrapped around me, I was ready to leave the hospital. The pink ladies escorted me out, needing a large tray to hold all the flowers, pillows, and other gifts I had received.

As I got into the car, my mother reached down and handed me the tie from my robe, which had fallen out the car door. It reminded me of a scene in *It's a Wonderful Life*, where George hands Mary the tie from the football robe saying, "Your tail, madam." Tears welled up in my eyes. I was happy to be out of the hospital, the surgery behind me, and on my way home.

My sister, Susan, who lives in Memphis, arrived that morning and began cleaning and preparing lunch for my return home. My mother left with a teary farewell, and as she stroked my face, she told me how proud she was of me.

As I settled into bed, Susan's first request surprised me. She wanted to see my new breasts. When I opened my gown, she was the first of many to proclaim, "They're beautiful. Dr. B. did a great job. They're better than mine." I wasn't quite ready to accept that since I hadn't really looked at them yet.

Susan was a good drill sergeant, directing the first of many care people I had hired from an agency to help with cleaning, driving, and other chores during my recovery. She was there, and that meant a lot to me.

The next day I received news about my pathology report from Dr. L.—it was not good. I had multiple sites of cancer in both breasts and ten of the twelve nodes removed came back positive for cancer. My emotions took a nosedive. I would get the full report the following week. I feared I would need radiation, and maybe more surgery. What if there was cancer in my left lymph nodes that had not been removed? What would happen next?

That afternoon Susan and I went to Dr. B.'s for a checkup. With some of the bandages on my belly removed, I looked down at it for the first time. The thin incision went from hip to hip, stretching across my now flat stomach.

Elaine helped me take my first "real" shower that evening—getting almost as wet as I did—it felt so good. Later, Susan faced one of her own fears. I was experiencing constipation from the surgery and the medications I was taking. When the cramps got intense I asked Susan to go to the drugstore just down the street to get me a stool softener. After much urging, Susan, who never went out alone after dark, let alone in a strange city, reluctantly left.

Just before my sister headed back to her home in Memphis, we sat back-to-back on my bed. I was already crying just thinking about what to say to her. I thanked her for coming to care for me. She said, "Blood is thicker than water, and you are my only sister."

Rhonda, my brother Eric's wife, took me for my checkup at Dr. B.'s. As I carefully walked in and sat down, another angel approached. She asked if I had just had surgery, saying that hers had been a year ago, and she was doing fine. I said I had ten of twelve positive nodes—she had had fourteen of nineteen and assured me I would be fine. My remaining three drains were removed, and I gave my body a closer look in the mirror. It didn't *feel* like my body anymore.

I was two weeks post-surgery, more mobile with less pain. I had completed my two weeks of antibiotic medication to prevent infection, but noticed the skin on my stomach was still red and thought it was from the recent surgery. Dr. B. had said all was okay during my recent visit—I had believed him.

With Robin accompanying me to Dr. L. for the results of the path report, I was extremely nervous due to the preliminary results he had given me. I needed all the support I could muster. My stomach had been hurting for a couple of days, but I just attributed it to the healing process. By the time we got to Dr. L.'s, I had terrible chills and could not get warm. Assuming it was a bad case of nerves, I asked for a blanket and was given a couple of paper gowns to wrap around me.

I sat in his office and the chills grew worse. I relied on Robin to get the details of my path report. Dr. L. expressed concern for an area close to my chest wall, suggesting radiation therapy. Although he deferred to Dr. G. for the continuation of my treatment, he mentioned a high-dose chemotherapy to treat advanced-stage cancer—stem cell transplant.

After returning home, I visited with my aunt Caroline who had arrived from Kansas to help. Unable to shake the chills, I went to lie down. Robin, in divine order, stayed and visited with my aunt. Still shivering under the blankets, I asked her to take my temperature—it was 104 degrees. With cold compresses on me, she called Dr. B.'s office. He ordered more antibiotics and Tylenol, saying to call the next morning if I still had a fever. I did.

Unfortunately, Dr. B. was in surgery and could not see me that day. His nurse, realizing how sick I was, got me an immediate appointment with Dr. C., an infectious disease doctor. I was dehydrated and very weak, so he sent me immediately to the ER for port access and IV antibiotic treatment. My temperature was still 104 degrees, and my heart was racing—antibiotics and fluids were quickly administered. When I experienced a burning sensation on my hands and face in reaction to the antibiotic, the IV flow was decreased.

Still dehydrated with fever, I was scheduled for IV antibiotic treatments throughout the weekend at the hospital's oncology infusion room. Arriving there in a daze, I remember thinking I was in a horror movie. The dingy room was filled with patients in chairs with bags of fluid in many colors hanging on poles. Nurses were running up and down tending to them. I waited for more than an hour to begin the treatment. I was feeling so sick, and so much commotion was going on around me that I just wanted to escape. With a slow drip, due to the previous night's reaction, I sat there, now a part of the horror show.

My friend Heather came to spend the night. I was still feverish and dehydrated. Mo, another support group friend, suggested I call the doctor to order fluids for my next IV treatment. Elaine recommended Gatorade for the dehydration and Imodium A-D to help the diarrhea I now had. Nauseated, I had not been able to eat for the past day or so. A protein drink helped, but it was another rough night. After three days of antibiotics and fluids, although still feverish, I felt better—the worst was over.

Robin spent that afternoon and evening with me. As we shared our life stories, we found our soul connection. Although we had led completely different lives, inside we were similar. She showed me compassion and spiritual guidance throughout my treatments. We continue to share a deepening relationship.

I needed IV antibiotic treatments daily, and a friend or relative acted as chauffeur. I was home alone, but I really was not alone. Love, support, prayers, and good wishes surrounded me each night, making me feel safe.

With most of my friends either out of town or busy with plans for the July 4th holiday, I still had two more days of treatment. Luckily, I found someone to drive me to the hospital. My own plans included an IV treatment, not barbecue and watermelon. I watched the fireworks on TV, not my idea of the way to spend the holiday.

After receiving my last IV treatment the next morning, I saw Dr. B. He had stuck a needle into my belly during my previous visit and withdrawn a great deal of fluid. It was sent to be cultured to determine the type of infection I had. Now he bounced around the exam room with relief, informing me that the infection was strep, but not the more dangerous strain that one can get while in the hospital.

Dr. G. recommended that I begin taking Taxol. We discussed other additional treatments, including the stem cell transplant. Dr. F., an expert on the subject, came in for a few minutes to talk to me. He felt that I might qualify for a research study using Taxol along with high-dose chemotherapy. He suggested we discuss it further, and an appointment was made.

If I chose the transplant, I would be under continuous treatment for the next five months. My research on the transplant was soon underway. After more than two weeks of daily doctor visits, I had three whole days without one. Yippee. This doctor stuff was really getting old.

July 7, 2000, I wrote in my journal:

I am going to die someday, so I might as well live until I do.

Do what I love and stay in touch with my feelings and desires. Accept my limitations and go beyond them. I can do more than I think I can. Remember the mountaintop—to see peace and beauty when I'm scared. I'm strong with the faith and love that is within me. Angels are always near to help me—accept and be open to them. Cry if I must, but remember to laugh too. Make my song heard with my actions. Give with an open heart. Be totally focused on each person I meet. Everything is provided in the now, so be present. Thoughts create the future. The past is only a memory—good and bad. Love is all there is—let it out. Use Robin as my role model, because this is who she is.

A month after surgery was the first time that DJ and I were intimate again. He was afraid to touch me at first, because he did not want to hurt me. His gentleness comforted me. As he began kissing me, I realized I had missed his touch, but when we moved into the bedroom I found I was not ready. He gently explored my new body, kissing both my breasts, asking how I felt, and if he was hurting me. I got the answer I needed—he still loved me, and was still sexually attracted to me.

Robin helped me research the stem cell transplant procedure. The latest studies showed that it did not affect the recurrence rate one way or the other. However, since my prognosis was of such a high-risk nature, I was willing to look at everything.

Robin was with me the morning of my first Taxol treatment. I had lost twenty pounds over the previous six months due to nausea, surgery, and infection. I asked that my dosage of Taxol be double-checked since it was calculated by weight. A correction was made, and my treatment proceeded.

As we left Dr. G.'s office, another angel appeared. Overhearing us discussing the stem cell procedure, she said that she had had it five years ago and was doing fine. Having had seventeen of seventeen positive nodes, she said she would do the procedure again, if her cancer returned. Her husband, who had since died, had helped her through the entire procedure.

My first experience with driving again came six weeks after surgery when I attended a church pre-camp meeting to teach photography to children. The camp director, aware of my situation, could not have been kinder. I looked forward to creating joy once again in my life as I passed my skills on to the children. Although the week was physically demanding, it was fun playing and shooting pictures with the kids. I was back in the real world again.

During that week Dr. G. had called to express her concern that my recent blood work showed an elevated cancer marker. When the doctor calls, alarms go off. She wanted to order a bone scan to rule out the possibility of bone cancer.

A bone scan was relatively easy now that I had accustomed myself to having needles stuck in my arm. As I left the hospital, I saw Dr. L. on the elevator. He asked me to call him with the results. The bone scan came back "clean"—no cancer. What a relief.

New blood work showed that both my red and white cell counts had nosedived from the chemo. I was off of fresh veggies again and back on Neupogen shots, as well as Procrit, to help me through the next chemo rounds.

At my two-month follow-up with Dr. B., I got up the courage to ask him about sexual intimacy. Would "smushing" my breasts or belly damage my body? He said, "Smush away. You wouldn't damage anything now." I was relieved to hear that, since DJ and I now had had two unsuccessful attempts—I was ready to try again.

The next time DJ came over, we had a wonderful time. Still unsure about my body image, I asked him his thoughts about my breasts. "They are only skin. In fact, they're your own skin," he said. Again, I really appreciated him. He helped me through a very emotional time.

It seemed that everywhere I went I met women who were going through the stem cell procedure. I got more information, and the difficulties that went with it, but I continued to feel that it was the right thing for me. With Robin again at my side, we met with Dr. F. to discuss the details of the procedure. Then, a glitch—my insurance company agreed to cover the transplant, but only if I was under the care of another doctor, Dr. H. It was the end of August, and I had my third Taxol treatment behind me. The days following each treatment had been easy and side-effect-free—I was tired, but had no nausea or bone pain.

I met with Dr. H. We sat face-to-face, alone in his conference room, as he gave me his medical background and said that the isolation facility at the hospital had been built to his specifications. Unfortunately, my risk for recurrence was at 80 percent, but I was not eligible for any study. He said that if there was any problem with my insurance company not covering the transplant, he would appeal their decision.

He could not tell me if the transplant would prevent a recurrence any better than the regular treatments I had already had. He was honest about the time it would take my body to recover, one year to eighteen months. That was longer than I had anticipated. He was brutally honest about the danger of the procedure and its side effects. Throughout the two-month process I would need a caregiver around the clock. That person would drive me back and forth for treatment, be my cheerleader when I was too weak to care, and handle any medical concerns that might arise—a daunting task for anyone. Who could I turn to? There would be preliminary testing for extensive blood work, lung and heart tests, bone and CAT scans, and a bone marrow biopsy. He also recommended radiation therapy following the transplant. I was given a very thorough physical exam, and after a four-hour visit the preliminary testing was scheduled.

Back home I felt more confused and scared than ever before, but

was convinced that Dr. H. would see me through this difficult passage—I trusted him explicitly. Divine order was again in charge of
my destiny.

Beth and Alice from my support group offered their help, as did
Gayle. And how I appreciated it. I knew that I could not do this
alone. Secure in my belief that God continued to protect and guide
me, people came into my life when I needed them most. I was also
strengthened by the spirit of my paternal grandmother, who as a
young woman with a six-year-old child traveled by ship from Europe
in steerage, leaving all her family and friends behind, to join my
grandfather in America and start a new life.

The preliminary tests were underway—bone scan, CAT scan,
and heart test. Except for the needle sticks, I was becoming pretty
familiar with this hospital "stuff." Gratefully, the scans were clear of
any cancer.

I was still undergoing testing after Labor Day. I saw Dr. H. to
have my swollen neck and face checked, which I had assumed was
due to some reaction. He felt that I was okay, and I went on with the
testing.

Obtaining blood from my port was difficult, and I found myself
back in radiology again for another dye study—this port thing was
really getting to me. They found a blood clot at the end of the port,
which they treated with clot busting drugs that took care of most of
the problem. Then back to Dr. H.'s office for the lung test, and the
bone marrow biopsy that I would be sedated for.

I began lining up my support team that Dr. H. said I would
need. Believing that I could make this happen with my friends, I
called them, but found that there were not enough people able to
take on that much responsibility. I called my brother Bert in tears.
What would happen to me if I couldn't get the help I needed? He
suggested I look in the paper for paid caregivers and not worry about
the cost. Dr. H. told me that he would not start the process unless I

had a committed caregiver—he had never lost a patient, and I was not going to be his first one.

Through an agency, I hired two women, Dorothy, the night caregiver, and Carol, for the daytime hours. Dorothy had a nurturing nature and made me feel safe and protected during the worst of the side effects. She was my cheerleader. Carol, on the other hand, did the bare minimum for my care. But this was my team, and I was going to make the best of it.

On September 29, Carol took me for my first day of treatment. It was Rosh Hashanah, and for the first time in my life I was not able to go to services and pray—it felt weird. But I was comforted knowing that on this Jewish High Holy Day so many people were praying for me. The doctors had decided that I could skip my fourth Taxol treatment, but would receive Cytoxan.

Dorothy arrived on time that first evening. Although it would take some getting used to having someone in my house at night, I knew I would get through it.

By the third day I felt physically okay, but Carol was not as helpful as I had hoped. I cared for myself and prepared my own meals, swollen from fluid retention, but thankfully, not nauseous for a change. I was appreciative when others prepared meals for me.

Cytoxan was doing its job—blood counts, including platelets, were dropping. The Neupogen shots, given by Elaine twice a day, helped to bring my white cell count back up to have enough stem cells to harvest. This was the most important part of the procedure, because if I did not get enough stem cells, my body would not have enough to work with after the high-dose chemo killed everything off.

The first couple of weeks went well with minimal side effects. Carol and Dorothy settled into their jobs helping me, and I was adjusting to them being in my home. I began giving myself the morning Neupogen shot after watching Elaine for the past few months—I just did it, finding I could do what I needed to do when I needed to do it.

The catheter procedure was done at the hospital and hurt more than I expected. It was implanted for the stem cell collection, high-dose chemo treatment, and the daily blood draws. I had a tube hanging from the right side of my chest with three outlets that had to be flushed each day to prevent infection. I also had my first platelet infusion—my body was holding its own.

However, the next morning I awoke with blood in the catheter and a slight fever. I called the doctor and was told to go to the hospital to be checked. I received my first infusion of red cells, which took the entire day. By that evening I was an emotional wreck, unprepared for problems so soon. Sharon came by for a visit, and that lifted my mood.

Collection Day! At Dr. H.'s, I was hooked up to what looked like a dialysis machine, with one tube for blood going out and another one for its return. It took over four hours and once hooked up, I could not leave the machine. I was given more fluids that again caused retention. Lasix, a diuretic, helped my kidneys release the buildup. I was given more platelets. Nothing seemed to help the cold, deep chill I felt during the procedure. A second day of collection followed; even though enough cells had been collected during the first day, these were harvested for insurance.

Carol was useless, sticking her head into my room a couple of times to check on me. She sat with me for about twenty minutes, but only at the nurse's insistence.

Once the collection was completed, I saw Dr. H. to go over the next steps. Beth took notes to update my family and friends on the remaining and most dangerous part of the stem cell transplant. The plan was to begin on a Monday, when I would start receiving four days of a combination of three high-dose chemo drugs that would be infused continuously. Then I would receive the transplant of my collected cells, requiring a hospital stay.

With the chemo treatment, I faced complete hair loss again. For the past few months my hair had started to grow back, which might not seem like much in the grand scheme of things—but at least I had hair to shampoo. Because of chemo I now also had high blood pressure. Due to my family medical history, I was concerned, but medication brought it under control. Feelings of isolation and loneliness started to set in—all my support was not enough. Although, the weekend before the high-dose treatment began, family members came to visit, and they had a pleasant and calming effect on me.

At Dr. H.'s I was hooked up to the chemo pumps and fluid. The day went well, except when Carol had to be hunted down to receive the instructions for my care. Back at home, the afternoon was filled with calls and visits from family and friends.

More fluid retention caused me to gain five pounds in just a few hours—I was back on diuretics. Dealing now with the familiar side effects of chemo, the infusion routine continued: fluids, blood check, nurse and doctor visits, all supplemented by the ongoing challenge of dealing with Carol's lack of care.

On the fourth day, unexpectedly, I got very sick after the treatment and started vomiting. Medication to ease the nausea didn't work, so the doctor had me admitted to the hospital. There was a delay, though—no beds were available until later that day. When Carol and I arrived in my room, she announced that she was leaving. "Wait," I said, "you have two more hours of duty." She said she was no longer responsible for me once I was in the hospital and left. The next day I fired her.

I sat alone in my room not knowing what to do. The hospital staff settled me into the isolation unit. My visitors wore booties over their shoes and gowns over their clothes to protect me from any infection. My immune system, destroyed by the chemo, would have to completely recover.

Transplant Day! October 30. Dr. H., along with the other two doctors from his group, as well as nurses and support staff, filled my small room with white-coated people carrying my precious stem cells in three large syringes. As each syringe was injected through my catheter, they talked soothingly to me. Soon it was finished. After a quick exam, all the white coats left my room, and I was alone again.

The next morning I was released from the hospital. Although I was feeling much better, I didn't feel ready to leave. When my friend Babs arrived to take me home, she wore a starched white nurse's cap, large glasses with a fake nose, and a big smile. After all, it was Halloween.

November passed in a sedated haze of anti-nausea drugs. Roberta, my new care person, was the sweet, nurturing person I had hoped Carol would be. Each morning she drove me to Dr. H. for my checkup, while I struggled with the nausea, unable to eat solid food. I took short walks to keep up my strength, but mostly I sat on the couch and watched TV to pass the time, as calls, e-mails, and visits continued to comfort and inspire me.

During the second week post-transplant, I got a small infection and was back in the isolation unit at the hospital for five days. Thankfully, the infection was caught early, and did not cause much of a problem.

By late November, my catheter was removed, and I was using my port again for IV fluids and blood draws. Recovering nicely, I did not need any of the blood products post-transplant that I had been told I would need.

Eating solid foods came on Thanksgiving Day, almost thirty days after the transplant, thanks to Sharon and Elaine, who brought me portions from their family meals. I was feeling better each day and was slowly weaning myself off the anti-nausea drugs. The daily trips to Dr. H. were cut back to every other day, and then every third day.

By the beginning of December, I was completely off the anti-nausea drugs and no longer needed Dorothy's and Roberta's caregiving.

It was scary not having anyone with me at night. Although I had had a little difficulty getting used to Dorothy's presence at first, I now missed her and the security I had felt. Once off the sedating medications, I realized how drugged I had been, and was now able to drive myself again.

I celebrated my fifty-third birthday on December 12, and Dr. H. released me from his care that day—a wonderful birthday present. The nurse proclaimed I had "miraculously" made it through the procedure as I said my good-byes to the staff—they had walked with me through the whole ordeal. I still had a long way to go to regain my strength, but it was all downhill from here. Or so I thought.

In late December, Dr. G. checked me over and recommended beginning radiation therapy in early January. I did not want to hear that. The past couple of months had been the coldest in years. For weeks it stayed below freezing, and there were several snowfalls. I was alone now, isolated due to the cold and my weakness. Doctor visits and grocery shopping were the only times I ventured outside. It was much too cold to walk in the neighborhood, so I would drive to the supermarket in the mornings when there were fewer people around and I could walk down all the aisles for exercise. To protect myself during the cold and flu season, I was told to wear a mask whenever I went anywhere. I had not had a cold throughout my treatments, but lived in constant fear with my weakened immune system.

During December my friends were busy with the holiday season and their families, so my visitors were few and far between. It seemed each of them had some infection during the month and wanted to protect me from any exposure. I was grateful for their calls and concern, but felt very lonely and started to go into a mild depression due to the isolation.

I was given some suggestions on how to deal with the isolation and depression that winter. My brother Eric likened life to a movie, with each day a frame, some bad and some good. I was in the bad part of the movie now, but the good part was coming. Brian, a long-time friend, suggested the movie was more like moments in time—the past showing up in the early frames, the future in later ones, and the present was the frame showing today. This helped me gain a better perspective. I knew things would get better—I just had to keep going.

It was during that winter that I realized I needed to deepen my relationship with my mother. She had shown her love throughout the year, and I needed to tell her how I felt. So at the end of one of our almost daily telephone calls, I said, "I love you." This was something that had always been difficult for me to say. She responded in kind. Now each call ended with "I love you," either said first by her or me. It feels strange now when we *don't* say "I love you" at the end of our conversations.

January 1, I began taking tamoxifen, and would for the next five years. Possible side effects included hot flashes, night sweats, and weight gain, which I hoped wouldn't happen to me. However, a little weight gain wouldn't hurt—I was down to 108 pounds, and all my clothes were three sizes too big.

Robin brought a new breast-cancer friend into my life. Her name was Virginia, and we clicked right away. I watched her handle her treatments with determination and courage and was able to pass on some of my hard-earned experiences and advice. Another special person, Danny, came into my life during this time. He was an incredible role model—every time he called, he only wanted to hear how I was doing and refused to talk about his own struggle with cancer.

I was tired of treatment. It had been almost a year, and I was ready to get on with my life. Both Dr. G. and Dr. H. recommended radiation therapy, but my body was telling me not to do it. However, in my resolve to do whatever it took to ensure my health, I agreed to the treatment. One more thing I told myself that I could do—don't let the fear stop me.

My radiation oncologist, Dr. S., recommended radiation to both breasts and lymph areas, from my chest to just below my neck. It seemed like a lot of radiation to me, and I was fearful of the side effects. The simulation was long and uncomfortable. I was on the table with my arms above my head, bare-chested for more than two hours. There were black marks and small tattoos all over my upper body.

The morning of my first radiation treatment I awoke scared. It was not scheduled until 4:00 p.m., so I had most of the day to worry about it. I was on the table for forty-five minutes, extremely cold and uncomfortable, arms raised over my head for so long that they became numb.

Life continued along with my medical treatments. The roof leaked, the plumbing needed repairing, and there was an uprooted tree hanging over my driveway from the neighbor's yard. I took these things in stride as I dealt with my fears of radiation.

My platelet and white cell counts dropped, probably due to the radiation, but the treatments continued. I counted the days—four down, twenty to go. Pep talks from friends helped lessen my fears of radiation. I quit fighting and found I had more energy to deal with life—and life got better. The house repairs were underway, and I unexpectedly received a check to cover them, reminding me that all I needed would be provided by God, always. My photography business was generating income and inquiries. I learned to care for myself in a loving manner with good food, good friends, and peace in my heart.

Blood checks were twice a week as the radiation was impacting my platelets. There was a nurse I nicknamed "Little Mary Sunshine," who worked in the infusion room at the hospital. Through some of my darkest days during the stem cell procedure, she would sit and talk to me. Her smile and inner glow lit up the room. Now I was happy to sit and talk with her again while I waited for my blood test results. Treatment continued—ten down, fourteen to go. Thankfully, my skin showed no signs of rash or burning. Radiation temporarily stopped when my counts plummeted. My red cell count also dropped, and I was put on Procrit shots. The tiredness began to impact my life, but radiation resumed when my platelets and red cell count showed improvement. My platelets neared the danger zone again. It was becoming too much for me. With the ups and downs of low platelets and red blood cell counts, radiation was stopped again. Dr. G. suggested a blood transfusion. I consulted another doctor who said I probably had gotten all the benefit I would get up to that point. Because of the lag time, he recommended I stop the radiation. I agreed and met with Dr. S. to inform him of my decision.

With the treatments behind me, it was time to recover. Time to get back to work, and on with my life. By mid-March I was feeling better. I continued to get regular blood checks to monitor my low counts.

Right before the Passover and Easter weekend, I awoke with a swollen neck and head. What could *this* be? I was not under any treatment, and my port had showed no problems during my weekly blood draws. I had a photo shoot that afternoon and planned to leave the next morning for Birmingham, to spend Passover with my family. I struggled during the photo shoot—lightheaded, dizzy, and weak. I thought I put up a good front, but I didn't fool my assistant or my client.

When I got home I called the doctor, but with the Easter weekend approaching, no doctors were available. Reaching a nurse, she said to go to the ER. I felt I was okay, but one look at me by the ER doctor and I was put on an anti-clot IV. My port was found, once again, completely clotted, and the ER doctor told me that I had a life-threatening condition. I was admitted to the hospital that night. It was midnight when I called my mother to say I would not be coming for Passover. Not only had I missed the High Holy Days due to treatment, I would now also miss Passover with my family. I was shuttled back and forth to radiology to check the status of the clot. I was stuck repeatedly for blood and, overall, was absolutely miserable. The port had to come out.

The radiologist removed the port (I was sedated but awake) and found a problem with a vein—a stent was put in it to keep it open. Back in my room I suddenly had trouble breathing and felt my heart racing. A chest X-ray showed that the stent procedure was not the problem—it was caused by the anesthetic side effects. By the time I was released from the hospital three days later, the swelling was almost gone. The following week Dr. L. removed my stitches and explained the stent procedure. He was pleased with the good job the radiologist had done.

Dr. G. started me on Coumadin to prevent clotting. There were now weekly blood draws to check the drug's level and adjust the dosage as needed. The effects from the radiation still showed that my platelet and red cell count remained low.

In May, I had my six-month stem cell follow-up—blood work, bone scan, CAT scan, and lung testing were done. All the tests were normal, except for a minor change on the CAT scan. It was scarring from the radiation. Seeing Dr. G. almost weekly for blood work, my counts slowly returned to the low normal range. I felt stronger.

I had the entire month of June without one doctor visit. What joy! I began to feel normal again. July's blood work showed a slight increase on my tumor marker test, but Dr. G. said it was nothing to worry about. Each monthly visit continued to show slight increases, and by November when it was time for my one-year follow-up scans, my marker had risen above the normal ranges. My November scans, however, came back normal.

The following February Dr. G. began to worry. My tumor marker had continued to rise, and she suggested another series of scans to check things out. I became worried as well. I had a strong feeling that something was going on, but I did not want to believe it.

My eighteen-month follow-up scans were done in early May. After my bone scan, a spinal X-ray was done. I had not had to have one before. The next day, which was a Friday, Dr. G. telephoned. "I really hate to tell you this, but there is a spot on your spine and several very small spots on your liver. I'm scheduling you for an MRI."

My world came crashing down again. All I had done to prevent a recurrence—it had only been six months since my treatments had ended—now seemed to have not helped at all. I had watched two of my friends lose their battle with cancer; I was devastated.

With Pam at my side comforting me, I went through the two-hour MRI procedure, and afterward I was shown the spot on my spine. Dr. G. reviewed the results and recommended that I undergo radiation to my spine, immediately. The radiation oncologist recommended fourteen treatments in all—I agreed to get started that day.

I completed the fourteen treatments to my spine with no problems. I was taken off tamoxifen and put on Femara, a newer hormonal drug to treat my liver. Unfortunately, two months later, after a follow-up CAT scan, Dr. G. said the tumors on the liver had actually gotten larger! She then recommended that I begin taking Xeloda, an oral chemo drug. IV treatments of Aredia are now administered once a month to keep my bones strong. MRI and CAT scans will continue to monitor my progress.

*   *   *   *

I am now living with cancer—one day at a time, trusting in God's love and guidance. My gut still tells me I will not die from this disease. I trust my doctors and my support team, which includes the entire universe, to carry me down the path that God has chosen for me, in peace.

I will *live* until I die.

A Remembrance

In the spring of 2004, Sheryl lost her courageous four-year battle with breast cancer. We mourn, along with her family, the tremendous loss of our "sister," but celebrate who she was. A loyal friend to many, a person who loved giving of herself in community service to help others, especially children, and a passionate and talented photographer—her talent is displayed in the individual photos taken for this book and in the back cover photograph. Sheryl visually knew what would work without having her trained eye actually behind the lens of the camera as her photographer friend, Jeff, snapped the pictures.

We will miss her, but her legacy and spirit live on in her story, which she so willingly shared with those in need of comfort and inspiration. Her words will undoubtedly continue to touch lives.

The last line of her story reads, "I will live until I die." And she did.

AUTHORS' ACKNOWLEDGMENTS

BEVERLY FLOWERS

I would like to thank:

My mother, not only for the time she spent caring for me, but also for her unconditional love.

My husband, Roland, for his eternal love.

Aunt Hilda, Aunt Sis, Auntie, Aunt Helen, and Teenie for their emotional support.

Don Hartsfield for keeping our "secret." Ava Ablakatov for always being there for me.

I owe a special debt of gratitude to Brenda Moore for her time and help during my recovery.

Marian Price for her love and understanding.

Cheryl Dozier and Stan Willis for their love and concern.

All of the members of the Network of Hope for loving and supporting one another. The Wellness Community for being a place of refuge and care for cancer patients and their families.

All the medical professionals for every minute of their time to help me complete this journey to complete wellness.

Linda Brown for being invaluable in helping me complete this story.

BETH BUTLER

To my daughter and friend, Alison, with all my love and gratitude for being the light of my life. I could not have gotten through this without the love and support that she gave unselfishly.

My eternal gratefulness to my sister, Marian, for helping me face this difficult time in my life and for sharing the fears remembered from our mother's death. I pray that we never have to face this again.

A very special thanks to Dr. Michaela Caruso, my radiation oncologist, for her compassion and understanding. Her level of involvement and concern far exceeded the norm and made a difficult time a little easier.

My heartfelt gratitude to my doctors, Dr. Steven Sanders, Dr. Pradeep Jolly, Jill Bowen and the chemo nurses at Georgia Cancer Specialists for always being concerned, professional, and most of all, caring.

To Rick, my thanks for all he did to help me keep the farm going when my energy level couldn't keep up, and for hanging in there with me even when I know I was difficult.

Many thanks to Pam for taking time away from her family and busy professional schedule to spend time with me and help me through the rough spots.

I will always be grateful for the unquestionable support extended by my managers, Robin Main and Bob Storey, and my co-workers at Scientific Atlanta, who allowed me to maintain a productive life throughout treatment. They're the best!

A special thanks to my friend Phil for always being there for me and knowing what I needed without having to ask. I am honored to have him as a friend.

SELDEN McCURRIE

To God for His many blessings.

My husband, Sam, whose love, support, and sense of humor make anything seem bearable.

Dr. C. M. and Barb, whose keen eyes saved my life. "Thank you" seems so inadequate.

Dr. D. R., for his compassion and patience.

My family, whose constant prayers and steadfast faith continue to sustain me.

Ann and Don S., special thanks for your prayers and love.

Peg S., thank you for your enduring friendship.

Ann C., who has done so much for me these past thirty-two years.

E. Alton C., for his kindness and the much appreciated work on my behalf.

Lisa C., who can always make me laugh.

Peggy M., thank you for listening and going above and beyond the call.

My fur family, thank you for choosing us.

The Wellness Community, for being a haven for cancer patients.

ROBIN McILVAIN

Love forever and always to my husband, David, who has not only remained by my side with his love and unending support for over thirty-six years of marriage, but ever since we became high school "sweethearts."

To my son, David, and daughter, Christy, who have blessed my life with unending joy and pride and my three precious grandchildren.

Though I am separated by many miles from my sisters, Sharon and Traci, and my brother, Gig, we remain close in heart. The same holds true for my other family members.

Through the years, I've been blessed with many special friendships—I cherish each and every one of them.

To Sandy Knebel, the best friend in the whole world.

My deepest gratitude to the following doctors and their staff for providing excellent care, compassion, and understanding: Dr. John Donnelly, Dr. Elizabeth Steinhaus, Dr. J. Bancroft Lesesne, Dr. Michela Caruso, Dr. Colleen Austin, Dr. Sharon Tinanoff, Dr. William Fortson, Dr. J. Patrick Luke, and Dr. David Greenstein.

To the staff at Northside Hospital in Atlanta, Georgia, where I have always received the finest care.

Special thanks to Dr. Jan McBarron, who as a board-certified doctor has taught me so much about my medical conditions, nutrition, and vitamin supplementation.

Appreciation to Robbie Burney and Jennifer Pearson for teaching me how to manage my lymphedema.

To Barbara Squires, who taught me so much about traditional Chinese medicine while helping me manage chronic pain through acupuncture.

Mary Drew began the journey of this book with us and shared its vision. We became soul mates. A strong warrior, she fought her breast cancer with enormous strength and courage. Her guiding spirit has watched over our book, even during the most challenging times.

There will always be a special place in my heart for all the extraordinary women I have met through my support group, including the coauthors of this book. We share a common bond, connecting our souls.

MARION HORTON

My husband, Claude, is my dearest friend, my lover, confidant, the father of my children, my sweetheart forever, so he has to be the first I thank for his support.

My father influenced me by insisting I could do anything I wanted to. My mother always cheered, even if we lost the game.

Sometimes I hesitate to thank doctors publicly, assuming they are doing their job, but Dr. Elizabeth Steinhaus and Dr. Richard Bardwell are both outstanding. They stand out among doctors because of their compassionate nature and their very caring ways. I am especially thankful.

I can always depend on my children, Steve, Craig, Melanie, and Matt. As we age they seem to want to do more for us. As for the grandchildren, it was Suzanne who helped me with the computer aspects of this endeavor.

My sister, Dolores, and my brother, Dick, are the very best. I can depend on either for anything.

I have many friends, good neighbors, and caring relatives, but there are two groups of friends who are very special: The Encouragers Bible Class that I teach at Roswell First Baptist Church whose members are always there for me with prayers, food, and their presence. My Sisters in Plastic (SIPS) are both generous and loving, and not just in times of trouble. There are twelve of us who are former Tupperware distributors or Tupperware executive managers. Opal Scott, at the age of seventy-five, with more than forty years in the business, is still active. What would I do without them?

As my story details, I shall forever be indebted to Carol Cohen.

Most importantly, I thank my God, who sent His Son Jesus to ensure my life in eternity.

ALICE COTTER FELDMAN

My husband, Ron, and I had a year of medical challenges that had to be met. We did not do it alone. A complete list of thanks would fill pages. I can only say that "thank you" is inadequate for the gratitude I hold for all my family and friends. Their love, prayers, and constancy gave me a solid foundation on which to stand.

My surgical, oncology, and radiology teams were superb. They were efficient, skilled, punctual, thoughtful, and ever interested in my care—my thanks to all of them.

Special appreciation must go to Ron, whose steadfast loyalty in the face of continuing crisis was the bedrock of my recovery. His love, concern, humor, and gentle care helped me through the difficult, dark days.

I thank the leaders and members of my support groups. No one knows how "it" is unless they have "been there and done that!"

Finally, I thank God for the generous gifts of love He bestowed on us.

Strength, patience, caring, and a return to a spiritual self has enhanced our lives. Life is good!

ELENA TILLÁN SANTAMARIA

Heartfelt thanks for the abundance of love, support, encouragement, and prayers that I received from my wonderful family and dear friends.

To my children, Jaclyn and Danny, who are my life. Through them, I found the strength to carry on, not to give up when I was at my weakest. I am so proud to be their mom.

To Bert, who will always have a place in my heart.

My gratitude for my mother, Carolina, who taught me how important it is not to lose faith and never to give up. And to my father, Jose, who watches over me from above. I thank them for their unconditional love.

To my excellent team of physicians who not only take care of me physically, but emotionally. Special appreciation for Dr. J. Patrick Luke, Dr. Iqbal Garsha, Dr. Franklyn L. Elliott, Dr. Jose Garcia, Dr. Peter Gutschenritter, and Dr. Colleen Austin.

Thanks to Dr. Edward F. "Buzz" Stringer III for his guidance in helping me make the right surgical decision.

I applaud the tireless dedication of all the scientists who are working to find a cure.

My grateful appreciation to the competent and compassionate staff of Northside Hospital in Atlanta, Georgia, who continue to extend their support and love to this day.

Northside Hospital's Network of Hope is a shining example to women that they, too, can embrace life after breast cancer.

My sincere gratitude to The Wellness Community-Atlanta, where I found an oasis of support and help.

I want to acknowledge all the cancer patients, their caregivers, and families whom I have had the privilege to meet as a Patient Advocate at Northside Hospital. They continue to touch and enrich my soul with their courage and determination to live. I honor those who lost the battle with this life-shattering disease. They are all truly heroes.

LORNA GOLDSTEIN

To the various medical teams in each city where I was treated for my cancer problems, my heartfelt thanks. I thank the myriad support staffs everywhere. It takes special people to work each day with those afflicted by this horrible disease.

I am indebted to Drs. Stanley Heisler, Lance Perling, and Eva Arkin for their early detection of my occurrences.

To Dr. Dan Dubovsky, my medical oncologist and quarterback in Atlanta, and Dr. Maria Theodoulou at Memorial Sloan-Kettering in New York, bless them for their ongoing support.

I gratefully appreciate The Wellness Community in Atlanta, and Hope and Cope in Montreal for their many special ways of helping cancer patients and their families.

To my family and friends. They are my mainstay to face each day with joy and thankfulness.

George, my love, my rock, and greatest fan. After more than forty years of marriage, we continue to think as one. His love and devotion keep me strong. I am looking forward to the many adventures still to be traveled.

ALICE ROLLO

Without my husband, John, at my side I could not have made it through the past few years.

My children and their spouses, Renee and Mike Fain, Greg and Suzanne Rollo, Delaine and Tim Barker; all of them mean so very much to me, and I deeply appreciate their love, prayers, and many phone calls.

I thank Dr. Melvin Abend for being such a wonderful surgeon and taking such good care of me through three surgeries.

Dr. L. Franklin Elliott II, who gave me a new breast and made me feel like a complete woman again.

My employers and fellow employees at Roswell Obstetrics/Gynecology—I cannot thank them enough for their support and prayers.

My sister, Nancy Carter, the best sister anyone could ever have. I am grateful for all her loving care and prayers.

My Sunday school class. Thanks to all of them for their love, support, prayers, cards, and many meals.

SHERYL SIEGEL

To the community of breast-cancer survivors without whose support this journey would have been much more difficult—my deepest thanks.

To my mama; mere words cannot express my love for her—I honor her loving spirit.

To my siblings, Susan, Bert, Eric, and Lennie, whose deeds and loving support cannot be measured in human terms. I will be forever changed by their compassion and nurturing love.

I thank with all my love, my sisters-in-law, Toby and Rhonda, for their listening ears and encouraging words that helped me through some of my toughest days.

My love and gratitude to the other members of my immediate and extended family for their love and support—Harold, Dana and Laurie Brooks, Carolyn Rubin, Herbert and Faye Miller, Bernard, Eline and Randall Edelstein.

A special friend and soul mate, Pam Landry, gave me gentle encouragement and loving strength, and saw me through many trials.

Robin McILvain, my other soul mate, offered unlimited love and compassion and showed me what life really is about.

My appreciation to Heather Barbour, who kept me focused on the joy of life.

Thanks to Sharon Samford, who reminded me that life is all about family.

I thank Jeri Gurley for her friendship and for bringing Fannye Brown into my life, who inspired me with her ongoing cards and phone calls.

To Bea Wallins, Gerri Phillips, Gayle Page, Babs Johnston, Lya Sorano, Betsy Cenker, Anita Stein, Elaine Taylor, Lyn Vangsnes, Bev Greenwald, Beth Butler, and Debra Albin, who impacted my life in many ways.

Special thanks to my doctors and their staffs—Dr. Janice Gallenshaw, Dr. Patrick Luke, Dr. Henry Holland, and Dr. Phillip Beegle.

I'm deeply grateful to the members of Congregation Beth Jacob for donating blood and platelets on my behalf.

In memory of Virginia Van Valzah and Danny Miller whose bright souls now rest with God.

THE WELLNESS COMMUNITY

The Wellness Community is the largest program in the United States devoted solely to providing cost-free services of psychological and social support to cancer patients, their families, and friends. It was founded in 1982 by Harold H. Benjamin, Ph.D., in Santa Monica, California. Since then, the program has spread to more than twenty locations across the nation and has delivered unique and extremely effective programs of psychosocial support, education, and hope to more than 35,000 people fighting for recovery from cancer. All programs are facilitated by licensed professionals. All programs are offered as added and complementary resources for participants to use as an adjunct to medical treatment.

One of Harold Benjamin's basic concepts is of the importance of being a "patient active." Clinical studies confirm the accuracy of his view that "cancer patients who participate in their fight for recovery along with their health care team will improve the quality of their lives and may enhance the possibility of their recovery." Every aspect of The Wellness Community provides an opportunity to be an active participant in the recovery process.

From the moment one walks through the door of the home-like setting, one feels a sense of being in a place of caring, learning, and growing with others. Benjamin believed that no one should have to face cancer alone. Newcomers are welcomed and are invited to join an ongoing **Participant Group** or **Family Group** in which people with cancer can create an extended family and explore new ways to deal with stressors and cancer. There are classes that facilitate new ways to respond to chronic stress, which clinical studies confirm to be an inhibitor of the immune system. **T'ai Chi** and **Interactive Yoga** provide gentle exercise as well as a sense of inner calm and well-being. A class in **Stress Reduction** explores techniques such as relaxation and visualization to enhance the immune system, to manage stress and pain, and to manage the side effects of treatment. **Recovery Through Art** and **Exploring Dreamwork** are classes that help access repressed feelings and tap into one's deep resources of wisdom and creativity. **Meditation** and **Survivorship** offer another doorway into inner resources for strength in the recovery process. Another class, **Spirituality and Cancer** explores cancer's impact on one's search for meaning.

Networking Groups are drop-in groups led by licensed psychotherapists where individuals can share common issues, information, and experience. They give participants an opportunity to connect with others who have the same type of cancer. Each month there are **Special Events** where experts on many topics offer information and facilitate dialogue on specific areas of concern. Programs on chemotherapy, pain management, nutrition, and mind-body connection are examples of the large variety. These programs aid participants in making informed, responsible choices for their own recovery process.

The Wellness Community is a place of fun and laughter. Each month there are parties and **Social Events** in which participants can relax and enjoy the company of family and friends, old and new.

The Wellness Community is a place of acceptance and comfort. It is a true community of hope and support. Participants may gain new perspectives and attitudes both toward illness and toward wellness. Priorities and expectations may expand and shift. A growing awareness of deep connection may spark new possibilities and purpose. As consciousness of outer resources grows, one may learn to be a true partner with one's health care team. As consciousness of inner resources grows, one may find an expanded sense of meaning and claim the reality of the richness and wholeness of life.

For locations and information, visit:
www.thewellnesscommunity.org

GLOSSARY

Adriamycin: A chemotherapeutic agent; one of the strongest drugs available.

areola: The dark area of skin that surrounds the nipple of the breast.

autologous stem cell transplant: A procedure in which bone marrow is removed before receiving high-dose chemotherapy and restored in the same person following intensive treatment.

axillary lymph node dissection: Removal of lymph nodes under the arm.

benign: Not cancerous.

bilateral mastectomy: Surgery to remove both breasts.

biopsy: The removal of tissue for examination under a microscope.

bone marrow biopsy: The removal of bone marrow tissue, using a needle, for examination under a microscope.

bone scan: A test to learn if cancer has spread to the bones.

brachial plexus: A network of nerves in the armpit, which go on to supply the arm.

breast prothesis: An artificial breast worn by women who have had mastectomy without reconstruction.

breast reconstruction: Surgery performed by a plastic surgeon to create an artificial breast after a mastectomy.

calcifications: Small calcium deposits in breast tissue that can be seen by mammography.

CAT (computerized axial tomography) scan: A series of detailed pictures of areas inside the body, at different angles.

chemotherapy: The use of certain chemicals to treat cancer.

comedo: Type of DCIS in which the cells filling the duct are more aggressive looking.

compression sleeve: An elasticized sleeve worn to manage lymphedema.

costochondritis: A type of arthritis that causes inflammation where the breastbone and ribs connect.

coumadin: A blood-thinning medication to prevent blood clots.

cribriform: Type of DCIS in which the cells filling the duct have punched out areas.

Cytoxan: A chemotherapeutic agent.

Decadron: A synthetic steroid used during chemotherapy treatment to decrease inflammation and swelling.

DNA: Short for deoxyribonucleic acid. A complex molecule containing the genetic information for inheritance.

ductal carcinoma in situ (DCIS): Also called intraductal carcinoma; ductal cancer cells which have not spread outside the duct to other tissues in the breast.

edema: Swelling caused by excess fluid in the soft tissues.

endometrial cancer: Cancer of the uterus that starts in the lining of the uterus known as the endometrium.

epirubicin: A chemotherapeutic agent.

Femara: An oral hormonal chemotherapy drug.

fibromyalgia: A rheumatic disorder characterized by pain, tenderness, and stiffness of muscles and connective tissue structures.

5-fluorouracil (5-FU): A chemotherapeutic agent.

frozen section: The freezing and slicing of tissue to expedite a diagnosis.

HER2/neu: A gene for the epidermal growth factor receptor; receptors make cells grow. If present, cancer cells may grow uncontrolled.

infiltrating cancer: Also called invasive cancer; it is a cancer that has grown beyond its original site into surrounding tissue.

Kytril: A drug used to control the nausea and vomiting associated with chemotherapy.

lumpectomy: Surgery to remove a cancerous lump with a small amount of normal tissue surrounding it.

lymphedema: A condition in which excess fluid collects in the tissue and causes swelling of the arm as a result of surgical removal of underarm lymph nodes. It can also occur following surgery and radiation without lymph node removal. This condition is not curable but is manageable with proper therapy by a licensed lymphedema therapist.

lymph nodes: Small, bean-shaped glands found in the body that help protect against foreign invaders, such as bacteria. Cancer can spread to the lymph nodes through the bloodstream and be carried along to other sites.

malignancy: Uncontrolled growth of cancerous cells.

margins: The removal of normal surrounding tissue in cancer surgery. "Clean" margins mean no cancer cells are found at the edge of the tissue, suggesting all of the cancer has been removed.

mastectomy: Surgery to remove the breast.

metastasis: The spread of cancer from one part of the body to another.

methotrexate: A chemotherapeutic agent.

modified radical mastectomy: Surgery to remove the breast, most or all of the lymph nodes in the armpit, the lining over the chest muscles, and sometimes part of the chest wall muscle.

necrosis: Dead tissue.

needle biopsy: The removal of tissue or fluid using a needle to aspirate for examination under a microscope.

nuclear grade: An evaluation of the size and shape of the nucleus in tumor cells and the percentage of those cells in the process of dividing and growing.

Nuepogen: A drug used during chemotherapy to increase the white blood cell count and to decrease the chance of infection.

pathology report: A report of the microscopic examination of cells and tissue.

port-a-cath: Also called a port. An implanted catheter through which blood can be withdrawn and drugs infused without repeated needle sticks.

proliferation: The multiplying of cells.

radiation therapy: High-energy radiation to kill cancer cells.

recurrence: The return of cancer after treatment to the same site as the original tumor or in another location.

sentinel lymph node biopsy: The removal of the sentinel lymph node(s) to which cancer cells are likely to spread.

S-phase fraction: A measure of cell division and growth of a tumor. If high, it can be an indicator of a more aggressive tumor.

stereotactic core biopsy: A minimally invasive procedure which uses a computer-guided core biopsy needle to drill a core of tissue.

tamoxifen: An oral estrogen blocker prescribed after breast-cancer treatment, usually taken for a five-year period. It is also prescribed as a preventive for high-risk women.

Taxol: A chemotherapeutic agent.

TRAM (transverse rectus abdominis muscle) flap: Procedure for breast reconstruction utilizing tissue and blood supply from the lower abdomen, below the navel.

Xeloda: An oral chemotherapeutic agent.

RECOMMENDED READING

Anderson, Greg. *Cancer: 50 Essential Things to Do.* New York: Plume, 1999.

Andrews, Ted. *Animal-Speak: The Spiritual and Magical Powers of Creatures Great and Small.* St. Paul, MN: Llewellyn Publications, 1993.

Armstrong, Lance. *It's Not About the Bike: My Journey Back to Life.* With Sally Jenkins. New York: G. P. Putnam's Sons, 2000.

Balch, James F. *The Super Antioxidants: Why They Will Change the Face of Healthcare in the 21st Century.* New York: M. Evans and Co., 1998.

Ban Breathnach, Sarah. *Simple Abundance: A Daybook of Comfort and Joy.* New York: Warner Books, 1995.

———. *Something More: Excavating Your Authentic Self.* New York: Warner Books, 1998.

———. *The Simple Abundance Journal of Gratitude.* New York: Warner Books, 1996.

Barasch, Marc Ian. *The Healing Path: A Soul Approach to Illness.* New York: G. P. Putnam's Sons, 1993.

Benjamin, Harold H. *The Wellness Community Guide to Fighting for Recovery from Cancer.* New York: G. P. Putnam's Sons, 1995.

Bernard, Jami. *Breast Cancer, There and Back: A Woman-to-Woman Guide.* New York: Warner Books, 2001.

Brinker, Nancy. *The Race Is Run One Step at a Time: My Personal Struggle—and Everywoman's Guide to Taking Charge of Breast Cancer.* With Catherine McEvily Harris. New York: Simon and Schuster, 1990.

Canfield, Jack, et al., comps. *Chicken Soup for the Surviving Soul.* Deerfield Beach, FL: Health Communications, 1996.

Chopra, Deepak. *How to Know God: The Soul's Journey into the Mystery of Mysteries.* New York: Crown Publishers, 2000.

Cousins, Norman. *Anatomy of an Illness as Perceived by the Patient.* Boston: G. K. Hall, 1980.

D'Adamo, Peter J. *Eat Right 4 Your Type.* New York: Putnam Pub Group, 1997.

Diamond, W. John, W. Lee Cowden, and Burton Goldberg. *An Alternative Medicine Definitive Guide to Cancer.* Tiburon, CA: Future Medicine Publishing, Inc., 1997.

Dyer, Diana. *A Dietitian's Cancer Story: Information and Inspiration for Recovery and Healing from a Three-time Cancer Survivor.* Ann Arbor, MI: Swan Press, 2000.

Estés, Clarissa Pinkola. *Women Who Run with the Wolves: Myths and Stories of the Wild Woman Archetype.* New York: Ballantine Books, 1992.

Fields, Danny. *Linda McCartney: A Portrait.* Los Angeles: Renaissance Books, 2000.

Finn, Robert. *Cancer Clinical Trials: Experimental Treatments and How They Can Help You.* Cambridge, MA: O'Reilly, 1999.

Greive, Bradley Trevor. *The Blue Day Book: A Lesson in Cheering Yourself Up.* Kansas City, MO: Andrews McMeel Publishing, 2000.

Hyde, Susan Sturges. *No More Bad-Hair Days: A Woman's Journey through Cancer, Chemotherapy, and Coping.* Atlanta, GA: Longstreet Press, 1996.

Issels, Josef. *Cancer, a Second Opinion.* New York: Avery Publishing, 1999.

Jordan, Hamilton. *No Such Thing as a Bad Day: A Memoir.* Atlanta, GA: Longstreet Press, 2000.

Justice, Blair. *A Different Kind of Health: Finding Well-Being Despite Illness.* Houston: Peak Press, 1998.

Kneece, Judy. *Your Breast Cancer Treatment Handbook: A Patient's Guide to Understanding the Disease, Treatment Options, and the Physical and Emotional Recovery from Breast Cancer.* West Columbia, SC: EduCare Publishing, 1995.

Kuner, Susan, et al. *Speak the Language of Healing: Living with Breast Cancer without Going to War.* Berkeley, CA: Conari Press, 1999.

Kushner, Harold S. *When All You've Ever Wanted Isn't Enough.* New York: Summit Books, 1986.

———. *When Bad Things Happen to Good People.* 2nd ed. New York: Schocken Books, 1989.

Lerner, Barron H. *The Breast Cancer Wars: Hope, Fear, and the Pursuit of a Cure in Twentieth-century America.* New York: Oxford University Press, 2001.

Lerner, Michael. *Choices in Healing: Integrating the Best of Conventional and Complementary Approaches to Cancer.* Cambridge, MA: MIT Press, 1994.

Lindbergh, Anne Morrow. *Gift from the Sea.* New York: Pantheon, 1955.

Love, Susan M. *Dr. Susan Love's Breast Book.* 3rd ed. With Karen Lindsey. New York: Perseus, 2000.

Lunden, Joan. *Wake-Up Calls: Making the Most Out of Every Day.* New York: McGraw-Hill, 2001.

McCarthy, Peggy, and Jo An Loren, eds. *Breast Cancer? Let Me Check My Schedule!* Boulder, CO: Westview Press, 1997.

Myss, Caroline M. *Why People Don't Heal and How They Can.* New York: Harmony Books, 1997.

Nash, Jennie. *The Victoria's Secret Catalog Never Stops Coming: And Other Lessons I Learned from Breast Cancer.* New York: Scribner, 2001.

Olsen, Cynthia B. *Essiac: A Native Herbal Cancer Remedy.* With contributions by Jim Chan and Christopher Gussa. Pagosa Springs, CO: Kali Press, 1998.

Pearson, Carol S. *Awakening the Heroes Within: Twelve Archetypes to Help Us Find Ourselves and Transform Our World.* San Francisco: HarperCollins, 1991.

Radner, Gilda. *It's Always Something.* New York: Simon and Schuster, 1989.

Raz, Hilda, ed. *Living on the Margins: Women Writers on Breast Cancer.* New York: Persea Books, 1999.

Redfield, James. *The Celestine Prophecy: An Adventure.* New York: Warner Books, 1995.

———. *The Celestine Vision: Living the New Spiritual Awareness.* New York: Warner Books, 1997.

———. *The Tenth Insight: Holding the Vision.* New York: Warner Books, 1996.

Reeves, Paula M. *Women's Intuition: Unlocking the Wisdom of the Body.* Berkeley, CA: Conari Press, 1999.

Remen, Rachel Naomi. *Kitchen Table Wisdom: Stories that Heal.* New York: Riverhead Books, 1996.

———. *My Grandfather's Blessings: Stories of Strength, Refuge, and Belonging.* New York: Riverhead Books, 2000.

Ruiz, Miguel. *The Four Agreements: A Practical Guide to Personal Freedom.* San Rafael, CA: Amber-Allen Publishing, 1997.

Schuller, Robert. *Life's Not Fair, but God Is Good.* Nashville, TN: Thomas Nelson, 1991.

Siegel, Bernie S. *Love, Medicine, and Miracles: Lessons Learned about Self-healing from a Surgeon's Experience with Exceptional Patients.* New York: HarperPerennial, 1990.

Spiegel, David. *Living Beyond Limits: New Hope and Help for Facing Life-threatening Illness.* New York: Times Books, 1993.

Spingarn, Natalie Davis. *The New Cancer Survivors: Living with Grace, Fighting with Spirit.* Baltimore: Johns Hopkins University Press, 1999.

Stabiner, Karen. *To Dance with the Devil: The New War on Breast Cancer.* New York: Delacort Press, 1997.

Wadler, Joyce. *My Breast: One Woman's Cancer Story.* Reading, MA: Addison-Wesley, 1992.

Walsch, Neale Donald. *Bringers of the Light.* Ashland, OR: Millennium Legacies, 1995.

———. *Conversations with God: An Uncommon Dialogue.* New York: G. P. Putnam's Sons, 1996.

Weiss, Marisa C., and Ellen Weiss. *Living Beyond Breast Cancer: A Survivor's Guide for When Treatment Ends and the Rest of Your Life Begins.* New York: Times Books, 1997.

Zakarian, Beverly. *The Activist Cancer Patient: How to Take Charge of Your Treatment.* New York: John Wiley and Sons, Inc., 1996.

Zuck, Colleen. *Daily Word: Love, Inspiration, and Guidance for Everyone.* Emmaus, PA: Daybreak Books, 1997.

Zukav, Gary. *The Seat of the Soul.* New York: Simon and Schuster, 1989.